American Medical Association

Physicians dedicated to the health of America

Strategic Career Management *for the* 21st Century Physician

Gigi Hirsch, MD

Strategic Career Management
for the 21st Century Physician

Internet address: www.ama-assn.org

Additional copies of this book may be ordered by calling toll free 800 621-8335.
Mention product number OP208899.

ISBN 1-57947-001-7

BP37:99-467:3M:12/99

About the Author

Gigi Hirsch, MD, is Chief Executive Officer of MD IntelliNet, LLC. Following her training and Chief Residency in Internal Medicine at Brown University, Dr Hirsch practiced full-time Emergency Medicine for nearly five years. During that time she worked as a staff physician in a suburban community hospital, as an urgent care team leader at Harvard Community Health Plan, and as an attending physician and teacher at Brigham and Women's Hospital. Dr Hirsch's observations, experiences, and discussions with many colleagues in clinical practice drew her attention to the problems impeding the effectiveness, professional growth, and career satisfaction of physicians. Her growing interest in this area led Dr Hirsch to a psychiatry residency at Boston's Beth Israel Hospital. Upon completing this training in 1992, she mobilized the support of several chiefs of service, as well as the president of Beth Israel Hospital, and created The Center for Physician Development (CPD), an off-site program of the hospital.

In 1997, CPD spun off from the hospital and was established as an independent consulting firm called Gigi Hirsch, MD & Associates. Dr Hirsch, executive director of the company, established an international reputation for her expertise in the impact of the changing health care environment on physicians. In this context, a substantial portion of Dr Hirsch's time was devoted to career consulting, particularly to physicians interested in diversifying their careers beyond direct patient care. She has consulted to hundreds of physicians over the past five years, many of whom heard of her services through widespread media coverage (eg, the *Wall Street Journal,* the *Chicago Tribune,* NPR's *Marketplace,* and *All Things Considered,* among others) and from the American Medical Association.

Dr Hirsch was an Instructor in psychiatry at Harvard Medical School from 1992 to 1997. She has previously held appointments as instructor in medicine at Harvard Medical School and assistant instructor in medicine at Brown University. She is currently a member of the American Medical Association, the Academy of Occupational and Organizational Psychiatry, the American Medical Informatics Association, and the MIT Enterprise Forum.

Acknowledgments

To my father, for his unwavering support through all of the uncertainties of my own career transitions.

To those colleagues and clients who have so generously shared their perspectives, personal stories, and support. Their contributions represent critical building blocks for the development of MD IntelliNet.

And to Michael P. Scott, for his support, wisdom, and creativity in editing this book.

The following people made significant contributions to the publication of this book. Their efforts are both acknowledged and appreciated.

Carol Sprague
Senior Corporate Recruiter
Division of Employee Relations and
Placement
American Medical Association

Suzanne Fraker
Director
Product Line Development
Book and Product Group
American Medical Association

Jean Roberts
Managing Editor
Product Line Development
Book and Product Group
American Medical Association

Patrick Dati
Marketing Manager
Sales and Marketing
Book and Product Group
American Medical Association

Selby Toporek
Senior Communications Coordinator
Marketing Services
Book and Product Group
American Medical Association

Karla Powell
Freelance Copyeditor

Boston, 1999

Contents

Introduction

When I first began career counseling for physicians—back in 1992—I fully expected to find that the primary factor driving my clients to seek my services would be the demands managed care placed on productivity, reimbursement, administrative matters, autonomy, and the like.

For many who have sought my assistance, this was indeed the case. For them the practice of medicine represented a special "calling." They thrived on their privileged relationship with patients, the intellectual challenge, and the overall sense that they were making a real difference in the world.

However, as managed care reshaped the industry and their work lives, these physicians no longer felt effective or connected to their patients, and their professional satisfaction was rapidly eroding. They came to me to see if there was something they could do—anything—to revitalize their professional passion.

But for others the story was not so simple. For them, managed care was only the tip of the iceberg. In fact, for many physicians, their present dissatisfaction with managed care masked a deeper, more long-standing dissatisfaction with their career. For these physicians it quickly became apparent they had chosen not simply the wrong specialty, but the wrong profession.

They may have known this for a number of years—perhaps as far back as their premedical years. However, once they were entrenched in the rigid American medical training process, it was difficult—if not impossible—to modify their career path.

Things that other students commonly do—take a year off, change "majors" (ie, a different specialty track), or leave the field entirely—all were deemed highly irregular. So instead of risking the stigma of having second thoughts, many simply reconciled themselves to their choice of a career in medicine and forged ahead. In the days before managed care, the extrinsic rewards of the profession—status, respect, authority, financial compensation—often outweighed any lack of intrinsic satisfaction in the work itself.

But when managed care eroded many of those extrinsic rewards, those physicians who were fundamentally ambivalent about their careers in the first place decided that enough was enough. Whether managed care has caused heretofore unseen symptoms of career disenchantment or whether it simply has provoked a "preexisting" condition, it is a phenomenon that has triggered seismic shifts within the medical profession.

In the past, dissatisfaction with medicine was simply not openly acknowledged. But now such talk is commonplace among physicians. So in a way we have managed care to thank for bringing buried disillusionment and uncertainty into the light.

Because career satisfaction for physicians was simply assumed in the past, no information or resources to help physicians with career planning were really established. Consequently, there wasn't even a language or framework for issues relating to the management of physician careers.

This book is based on insights I've gained from more than 700 career consultations held with physicians since 1992. (All illustrations and case studies have been modified to protect confidentiality.) I hope it will help introduce that new language and framework, which in turn may help the medical profession move to a new level of sophistication and effectiveness in career management.

To my mind, this new era of open communication represents a tremendous opportunity for the entire medical system in the United States. By paying attention to the dissatisfactions of our peers, we may discover as a group how to foster healthy and successful career development of physicians at all life stages.

This book is not likely to add much value to the lives of those who find the practice of medicine today completely satisfying and who still believe in the traditional model of professional development. Additionally, those who have begun to recognize signs of career dissatisfaction may not be ready for this book if their disillusionment is recent.

Typically, physicians go through emotional stages when their dissatisfaction catches up to them, instead of being reflected on over time. The initial stage is often intense anger and/or grief. The intensity of these feelings often interferes with one's ability to absorb new ideas and suggestions for constructive actions. Again, this book may not be in the best interests of those at this stage of the process. Other resources exist that may be more helpful at this point, some of which are listed at the end of this Introduction.

This book is for those physicians who have moved beyond despair and are actively seeking options. It's for those who accept that no one else is going to rescue them or provide a ready-made answer. It is for those interested in learning creative ways to conquer the "new world" of health care.

This book is for those who are up to the challenge and excited about exploring a new sense of freedom in their career and their life.

References

Baker LC, Cantor JC, Miles EL, Sandy LG. What makes young HMO physicians satisfied? *HMO Pract 8.* 1994;No. 2:53-56.

Bloomberg MA, Mohile SR, eds. *Physicians in Managed Care: A Career Guide.* Tampa, Fla: American College of Physician Executives; 1994.

Chuck JM, Nesbitt TS, Kwan M, Kam SM. Is being a doctor still fun? *West J Med 159.* 1993;No. 6:1-3.

Dahl D. Rediscovering the joy of medicine. *Hippocrates.* November 1997.

Flower J. Job shift. *Healthcare Forum J.* January-February 1997.

Lewis CE, Prout DM, Leake B. How satisfying is the practice of internal medicine? *Ann Intern Med.* 1991;114:1-5.

Madison DL, Konrad TR. Large medical group-practice organizations and employed physicians: a relationship in transition. *Milbank Q.* 1988;66:240-282.

Pearson T, Haid RL, eds. The changing landscape of career development in medicine. *Career Plann and Dev J 14.* 1998;No. 1.

Pines A, Aronson E. *Career Burnout: Causes and Cures.* New York, NY: The Free Press; 1988.

Rutler T. Careers in crisis. *Harvard Med Alumni Bull.* Winter 1996.

Stamps PL, Cruz NTB. *Issues in Physician Satisfaction.* Ann Arbor, Mich: New Perspectives in Health Administration Press; 1994.

Wilson BA. Breaking away. *Unique Opportunities.* January-February 1997.

Chapter 1

The Issues

◢ A Changing Profession

The medical profession is in crisis. This crisis is not due to a lack of technology or treatments, nor is it due to a lack of physicians. This crisis is much more insidious. The crisis is burnout. Much of the blame for this prevailing malaise lies squarely at the feet of managed care—an economic and social experiment that has dramatically and irrevocably altered the landscape of American medicine. The results are staggering. Today's physician faces:

▼ A surplus of 100,000 to 150,000 physicians in the United States, many of whom are currently struggling to find nonclinical career alternatives.[1]

▼ A greater than 60% increase in the incidence of physician disability claims reported between 1990 and 1997.[2] Although the type of claim varies, the trend is fueled largely by the increased professional dissatisfaction of physicians. In the past, even if physicians had a legitimate disability, it was quite uncommon to file for disability. Rather, they would try to find some way to remain in medicine. Today, with the same impairment, they are much more likely to file a claim because they no longer want to be in medicine.

The costs for such dissatisfaction can be steep indeed—between $5 million and $10 million over the lifetime of the claim. (Associated costs are fueled by the notable challenge of finding viable career options for disabled physicians, which results in prolonged claim durations.)

▼ An intense pressure for earnings. As many as 90% of physician organizations in California are poised for bankruptcy or closure. More than 4,000 California physicians are owed an estimated $100 million following the bankruptcy of a major practice management company.[3] In addition, under many capitation contracts, 15% to 50% of payments to physicians are withheld until the end of

---

[1] Pew Health Professions Commission. *Shifting the Supply of Our Health Care Workforce: A Guide to Redirecting Federal Subsidy of Medical Education.* San Francisco, Calif: Pew Health Professions Commission; October 1995.

[2] Ainge D. Increased physician disability claims causing crisis. *MGM J.* September-October 1997.

[3] California Medical Association. *The Coming Medical Group Failure Epidemic.* San Francisco, Calif: California Medical Association; September 2, 1999:1. Special Report.

the year.[4] All of this is superimposed on an average medical school debt of $75,000.[5]

▼ A fourfold rate of increase in the incidence of physician suicide in the past two years in certain areas of the country with an unusually high penetration of managed care.[6]

The sad result of such statistics is that 30% to 50% of surveyed physicians report they would not choose a medical career if they had it to do over.[7]

For many physicians, these data provide some context for their own experience and help them understand they are not alone in their distress. However, numbers on a printed page do not begin to convey their difficulty in coming to grips with career dissatisfaction.

These days people change careers an average of seven times in their lives. If that's the case, why is it so devastating for physicians to realize they may want or need some type of career change?

How well physicians deal with career change is directly related to the initial expectations they had when they chose the medical profession. These expectations shape what is known as the "psychological contract"—the unspoken, and often unconscious, expectations physicians have of their work and the role it will play in their lives. If this psychological contract were a written document, it might read something like this:

> I agree to sign away approximately a decade of my life for my medical training with the guarantee that I will ultimately receive professional autonomy, respect, status, financial and job security, meaningful and intellectually challenging work, and career gratification.

The pervasive changes in medicine over the past 20 years or so actually constitute a breach of that psychological contract. Whenever there is a disruption in a psychological contract, it is met with the same sense of violation and betrayal that occurs when any type of contract is broken.

One's response follows a cognitive pattern that is somewhat similar to the grief-acceptance cycle formulated by Elizabeth Kubler-Ross, MD. Although an individual may not experience these stages in a clearly defined linear sequence, he or she is likely to experience at least some of the following elements (adapted with permission from Ralph Hirschowitz, MD).

---

[4] Greene J. Feeling the squeeze. *Modern Physician.* February 1998:48-50.

[5] *Managing Medical School Indebtedness from Educational Loans.* AAMC Fact Sheet; August 18, 1997.

[6] Personal discussion with anonymous source within a state Physician Health Program.

[7] Schroeder S. The troubled profession: is medicine's glass half full or half empty? *Ann Intern Med.* 1992;116:583-592.

Detachment

Impact. After the initial impact of change has registered, there is a disruption of the normal flow of the individual's life. At first he or she is stunned and may experience disbelief and an attempt or desire to carry on as if nothing has altered.

Disorganization. The individual enters a period of disorganization, marked by anxiety and a desperate attempt to reconstruct the world as previously known.

Reattachment

Recovery. During this period there is another series of cognitive and emotional processes, which help the individual break old attachments and reconnect with new ones. This is often the major work that allows individuals to adapt to change and then move on. During this phase, individuals may experience the following:

▼ *Disidentification:* Questioning one's identity, values, priorities, and relationships

▼ *Disenchantment:* Loss in belief system; puncturing of idealizations

▼ *Disorientation:* Confusion, loss of old landmarks not yet replaced by new ones

Reorganization. A final coming to terms with the changes and a commitment either to move forward and adapt or to design a new plan for the future.

It is difficult for individuals in the detachment phases to absorb and process new information about career planning and management. During the impact phase, their denial precludes intake of new information. During the disorganization phase, they are resistant to change, clinging to what is left of the old.

Many physicians have difficulty moving into the reattachment phases. Factors that contribute to keeping physicians stuck in the detachment phases include:

▼ friends, family, and counselors imposing their values onto the physician, which only discourages full reflection on his or her professional identity;

▼ a sense of guilt about taking care of oneself and one's own destiny;

▼ a lack of information about new, successful methods of adaptation within clinical medicine;

▼ a lack of information about one's options (alternatives to the traditional clinical career for physicians);

▼ a lack of time, energy, and/or self-confidence to explore these options; and

▼ an inability to move past initial anger and bitterness.

This book is designed to help individuals get unstuck and to move into the reattachment phases.

◢ Beyond Managed Care

The phases noted above apply not only to our professional lives in the face of managed care. Indeed, they represent a useful model for thinking about change in all areas of our lives. A useful way of visualizing this is to refer to the following diagram of the key spheres in our lives that need to be attended to as we manage our careers. Together, these spheres form what we will refer to as the "career ecosystem."

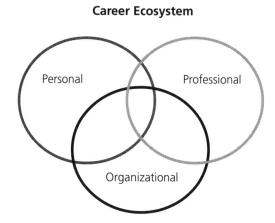

Applying the term *career ecosystem* to this concept emphasizes the complexity of the interrelationships among the three spheres which, together, function as a whole for each of us. When elements of one sphere shift, those of the other spheres necessarily shift too.

This schematic is a simple but useful tool for organizing and giving priority to issues that affect career satisfaction and effectiveness. We will take a closer look at this in Chapter 2.

Within each of these spheres, the most constant feature is change. Some changes are predictable; others are not. In some cases change is thrust upon us and is beyond our control. In other cases we may recognize the need for change and initiate it ourselves. In Chapter 2 we will explore how to manage change as a way of maintaining balance among these three spheres of our lives.

◢ Nothing Is Simple

Strategic career management is not a simple process. It's not just a matter of switching specialties or hospital affiliations. It's not running off to open a bed-and-breakfast. Strategic career management—and the key word here is *strategic*—is actually quite complex, with many interdependent elements—all of which will be discussed in upcoming chapters.

If you've begun to wonder, given the number of complex issues to be resolved, how anyone ever manages to achieve and maintain career satisfaction, don't give up yet. That's what this book will help you learn.

References

Bridges W. *Transitions: Making Sense of Life's Changes.* New York, NY: Addison-Wesley Publishing Company, 1980.

Hudson FM. *The Adult Years: Mastering the Art of Self-Renewal.* San Francisco, Calif: Jossey-Bass Publishers, 1991.

Chapter 2

The Career Ecosystem

When I first began providing physician clients with career consultations, it was somewhat overwhelming to hear them talk about all of their concerns, frustrations, and uncertainties. The expression of their thoughts was chaotic, unprocessed, and often intensely emotional. However, it soon became evident that it was possible to organize their issues into three key areas. Each area was separate, yet also symbiotic with the other two. I began to think of them as "spheres of influence."

Once the physician's random thoughts and themes were dissected and grouped into these key spheres, it became easier to define which were primary issues, which were secondary, and how to give them some sense of priority and order.

However, what became clear about these three spheres of influence was that there was a significant interrelationship among them. They did not function in isolation. A major change in one sphere almost always resulted in a compensatory change in another, or in both of the others.

In addition, by observing patterns emerge in my clients' lives, I came to appreciate the importance of the interplay between the environment of the physician and the individual. This helped me to understand why I found so many discussions and writings about physician burnout to be inadequate. Historically, physician burnout is discussed primarily in reference to the personality traits and coping styles that are typical of physicians and that leave us particularly vulnerable to burnout. While there is certainly a great deal of truth to this line of thinking, it fails to explore important environmental factors that—in combination with traits intrinsic to the individual—have a tremendous impact on career satisfaction. These environmental factors relate to the professional culture and organizational work styles that shape the world in which the individual lives, grows, and works.

It became increasingly clear to me that strategic career management demands that one understand the scope of these key spheres and the interrelationships among them. For together they function as a whole. Thus, we refer to the schematic that follows as a "career ecosystem."

Career Ecosystem

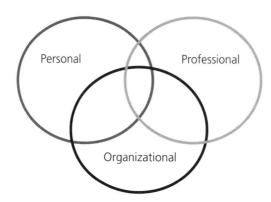

As a whole, the issues are complex. By teasing apart the various issues at play for an individual at a given point in time, planning and decision making become more manageable. This schematic is designed to provide a basic tool to facilitate this process.

Overall, I found that being able to give my clients a simple, rational, and organized framework for assessing the issues they were facing gave them some immediate relief. It also gave them a sense of empowerment and hope.

The *personal* sphere encompasses the following issues:

▼ The individual's physical and psychological health, plus that of close friends and family

▼ Quality of relationships with friends and family members

▼ Financial security

▼ Life transitions (eg, marriage, parenthood, caring for aging parents)

Example

A 38-year-old pediatrician has just been diagnosed with multiple sclerosis and wants guidance about how to modify her current work situation, as well as how to plan for the future of herself and her family.

She wants to cut back to a part-time clinical position in her HMO and find other nonclinical ways of using her expertise. This will enable her to make a transition to work that is more flexible and less stressful.

Furthermore, she is willing to pursue further academic training now, if the additional skills and credentials would enhance her future career options. She is fortunate to have no financial concerns during this process because her husband generates a lucrative salary.

In this case, the primary problem lies in the personal sphere, but it is also triggering active changes in both the professional and organizational spheres.

The *professional* sphere encompasses the following types of issues:

▼ Achieving and maintaining mastery over the physician's areas of technical expertise

▼ Relationships with both patients and colleagues

▼ Overall sense of satisfaction with professional life as it relates to such things as personal identity, values, and goals, as well as to spiritual aspects of work

▼ Malpractice stress

▼ Professional development opportunities

Example

A 42-year-old psychiatrist is bored with full-time clinical practice and wants to leverage the skills he has gained in his psychotherapy practice. He is wondering how he might diversify his professional activities to include the coaching of executives in corporations, as well as organizational consulting.

He currently works in a solo private practice. He has two children in Ivy League colleges. In this case, the primary issue lies within the individual's professional sphere.

However, helping him achieve his new professional goal is a challenge because of several key factors in the personal sphere (substantial cost of tuition for the next few years, for instance) as well as the organizational (how to find the time as a sole practitioner).

The organizational relates to features of our work environment that affect our ability to deliver safe, high-quality care to patients, as well as maintain balance between work and private life. The *organizational* sphere encompasses the following issues:

▼ Administrative policies and procedures

▼ Incentives and reward systems

▼ Decision-making processes

▼ Physical layout of office and/or work area

▼ Quality of support systems (ancillary staff, quality and extent of technology, etc)

▼ Access to career growth opportunities within the organization

Example

A 45-year-old primary care physician is increasingly frustrated with the lack of control over his daily work life within his staff model HMO. He is particularly frustrated with patient scheduling, which is done by an assistant who reports to an administrative supervisor rather than to him.

As his work stress increases, he becomes more short-tempered, not only with his staff, but also with his wife and children. By the end of each week, he feels emotionally depleted and is beginning to question whether he should leave clinical medicine altogether and find some other type of work.

In this case, the individual's key problems lie within his organizational sphere, but they also are negatively affecting his personal sphere. The overlapping problems in those two spheres further make him question his choice of medicine as a career (ie, the professional sphere).

◪ Case Study

Interplay Among the Spheres

Dr Jones is a 38-year-old internist working for a staff model HMO. Over the previous year, his organization has gone through a tremendous amount of turmoil and change. In addition to moving to a new location, the organization underwent a number of staffing changes. These included layoffs of 25 of its 150 employees, several changes on its executive management team, and the departure of two full-time female physicians who quit simultaneously because of perceived gender inequities in the organization.

Eight months ago, Dr Jones was promoted to medical director of the center. Although he had never before considered moving into management, he was flattered to be elected by his peers to do so.

Dr Jones received no formal training or mentoring in his transition to management. In addition, he was unaware of any professional associations that might have assisted him in attaining the skills and support necessary to perform effectively in this new role. He quickly began feeling overwhelmed with his new responsibilities and accurately sensed that he had minimal, and declining, credibility with physicians in the organization because of his ineffectiveness as a physician manager.

As his confidence in his management ability eroded, Dr Jones began to be concerned about how his performance would be assessed. Although he tried to discuss what evaluation parameters would be used to assess his performance, and at what time intervals, no one clarified this for him. Consequently he decided that, although only 25% of his time was to be spent in direct patient care, he would increase his productivity in that area because he knew he could do this well. He hoped that might compensate for any perceived deficiencies he demonstrated as a manager.

In short order Dr Jones was significantly overextended with his clinical responsibilities and began to feel unable to perform to his usual high standards with patients because of the time constraints dictated by his administrative role. At the same time, he continued to feel inadequate in managing his administrative responsibilities. His days stretched longer and longer into the evenings, allowing him less and less time with his wife and 3-year-old son.

Eight months into his tenure as medical director, Dr Jones described that things were in a crisis for him. "I feel like I'm having a nervous breakdown, and my wife is threatening to divorce me if I don't step down as medical director. I don't really know what to do. I am beginning to feel so stressed out that I even went to the Employee Assistance Program, but they didn't really seem to know how to help me. They had never worked with a doctor as a patient before."

This case study provides a rich illustration of the interdependence of the three spheres when a physician undergoes a major career transition. But more than being just one case study, it also provides a broader context for any individual's personal, professional, and organizational spheres of life. As is often the case for physicians, as well as for others, today's career management challenges result from changes occurring in the world around us.

For example, increased competition in the local or regional health market may unleash a cascade of changes that directly affect the shape and quality of an individual physician's daily work life. This was certainly the case for Dr Jones, where the initial changes began within the organizational sphere. The complexity and impact of this cascade of changes can be broken down as follows.

◢ Organizational Sphere

The HMO Dr Jones works for underwent massive changes in the previous year that included not only a move to a new location and facility but also substantial staffing changes.

Some of these staffing changes occurred by design, eg, planned downsizing and layoffs. But other changes were not planned. Consequently, the organization lost some of its pivotal employees when they became disgruntled with the HMO's management during a time of great transition and stress. In turn, the organization dealt ineffectively with the loss of key clinical people, as well as general understaffing, which resulted from unanticipated personnel changes.

In addition to the above personnel issues, the HMO clearly had significant problems resulting from real or perceived gender inequities within the organization. Left with only two remaining female physicians, access to care for those patients who prefer a female physician became another problem. In addition, the loss of two respected professionals from the staff lowered morale for the remaining women on the nursing and physician staff. Still, the HMO administrators denied any sex discrimination and blamed the problem on the "difficult" personalities of the two female physicians who resigned.

When establishing a medical director position, the many complex aspects of this job were poorly defined by the HMO. In addition, performance assessment tools were not as yet formulated. This lack of planning essentially doomed whoever was selected to almost certain failure. Dr Jones was flattered to be elected by his peers into this new leadership role, but was it in fact a good career move for him?

Dr Jones loved his clinical work and had never even considered moving into a management role. In fact, since he had never before worked in an organization that had a medical director, he had no idea what this role might entail. There were no former medical directors within the clinic site with whom he could discuss his decision. Unfortunately, he also did not know any medical directors working outside of his HMO, nor was he aware of any professional resources (eg, the American College of Physician Executives) that might have assisted him in this consideration. So his decision to accept the position was made pretty much in a vacuum.

Compounding the problem, the HMO did not provide adequate formal training to help Dr Jones move into this completely different role. Although the HMO's parent organization had periodic meetings for medical directors throughout its system, there was no formal curriculum for individuals making the transition to management. Again, it is unfortunate that neither the HMO, nor the other medical directors within it, apprised Dr Jones of the existence of the American College of Physician Executives, which provides just such a curriculum.

Although these critical components began within the organizational sphere, we will see their dramatic implications for Dr Jones' professional identity, as well as his personal quality of life. For example, when Dr Jones recognized the toll his new position was taking on him, he did what few physicians do. He turned to the HMO's Employee Assistance Program (EAP) for help. Unfortunately, EAPs in general tend not to have much experience or expertise in working with physicians as patients. This lack of support contributed to the stress associated with his career transition.

Professional Sphere

Although Dr Jones was initially very excited about his new management role, his growing sense of ineffectiveness soon made him yearn for the professional satisfaction he had always experienced in his clinical role. As for most physicians, his professional satisfaction was intertwined with his standards for personal excellence—an objective that seemed increasingly unattainable in his new management role.

Dr Jones' uncertain job security grew right alongside of his feelings of ineffectiveness in his new role. While it was unclear how the HMO intended to assess his performance and productivity as medical director, he did know he could excel in both those areas in his clinical role. So, as his anxiety about his performance as a manager increased, he added additional hours of patient care to his already long days. That way he did what he felt he could to increase his value to the organization. In other words, he reacted to stress in the way most physicians do: by working harder. Unfortunately, this did not address the fundamental issues that needed clarification in regard to his new management role.

Before taking the position of medical director, Dr Jones had enjoyed the collegial professional environment of his HMO. After starting his new job, he noticed a tremendous change in his peer relationships. He began to lose credibility with the other physicians, and he gradually felt ostracized and isolated. With no interaction among either administrators or physicians, Dr Jones' painful isolation added to his stress.

Personal Sphere

As Dr Jones worked harder, his availability to his family and friends, in terms of both time and emotional energy, was diminished. The quality of these relationships suffered over time, adding to his sense of failure. He knew he was letting the truly important people in his life down, but he did not know how to gain control over what was fueling this precipitous downward spiral.

In addition—because of the guilt his failing relationships caused and because, like many Americans, he didn't know how to cope with stress—he was unable to replenish himself emotionally and spiritually when away from work. As all of these factors overtook his life, Dr Jones said he began to think he was having "a nervous breakdown."

His health was becoming increasingly compromised, both physically and emotionally. Having lost his own personal physician—one of the two female physicians who had left the HMO—and with the EAP ineffective in assisting him, he felt more and more anxious about how to improve his life and his health.

◤ Complex Issues

The complexity of these issues, along with their interdependent dynamics, obviously makes them challenging to confront. There is a tendency to see such situations as simply the problems of one individual—in this case, Dr Jones. It's easy to dismiss them as evidence of poor leadership skills or difficulty coping with stress and change.

The conclusion drawn from this case could be that the organization selected the wrong physician to be medical director and that he should have been asked to step down so a new one could be selected. But without reflecting on the many lessons to be learned from this case, little will change. A willingness to learn from failed experiences could prevent the organization, not to mention Dr Jones, from experiencing unnecessary future failures.

◤ Predictable vs Unpredictable Challenges

Changes in medicine create new challenges, new stresses, and new opportunities, all within a very chaotic environment. Although the challenges we face today may be more dramatic than in the past, change is a constant of life. Some changes, like managed care, may have been unpredictable; but others are actually quite predictable. That's true of changes within the personal and professional spheres of our life as well (see chart).

Predictable and Unpredictable Changes

Sphere	Predictable Changes/Stressors	Unpredictable Changes/Stressors

Personal	Birth
	Marriage/Partnering
	Childbearing
	Terminal illness and
	  death of parents or
	  other loved ones
		Divorce
		Health problems

Professional	Entering medical school
	Residency
	Beginning practice
	CME
	Retirement
		Malpractice suit
		Professional role
		  redefined by
		  managed care
		Technology

And when changes in the personal sphere unfold—whether predictable or not—they have an impact on the stability of life within the professional sphere, and vice versa (see illustration).

The Constancy of Change

[Predictable] Professional

| Nursery School | Medical School | Residency | Practice | | Retirement |

Divorce Health Problem Managed Care

Unpredictable

[Predictable] Personal

Birth   Marriage Childbearing   Death of Parents   Death

Juggling change in your personal and professional spheres is challenging enough. But in the past 10 to 15 years, the organizational sphere has become ever more prominent for physicians.

Indeed, this sphere adds another full dimension of dynamic challenges to career management. Thus, whether the adjustment is to advancing technology, new leadership, or a merger, physicians must be prepared to cope with change within their organizational work environment.

It should be clear by now that achieving and maintaining a healthy, thriving career ecosystem is no easy feat. It requires ongoing attention and effort, which is richly rewarded when each new level of growth and restabilization is reached. The following story provides a wonderful illustration of this.

◄ Case Study

Professional Identity Crisis

This compelling illustration shows one physician's personal transformation, which led him to move beyond his professional identity as a surgeon. What follows is a series of e-mail correspondences that documents a pivotal phase of his career transition.

Dr G, a 52-year-old general surgeon approached my Web site while struggling with a career transition. He was unsettled from 10 years of ongoing family problems (wife with alcoholism, daughter with eating disorder) and the psychological counseling (family, marital, and individual) he underwent to help deal with these issues. He had also begun exploring Buddhism during this time.

July 1998

I have had major discontent with being a surgeon for at least 5 years or so because of the usual things—changes in our health care system, etc. But in the last few years—because of a shift in my personality and my new focus on listening, compassion, and caring (as opposed to the stereotypical surgeon's traits of technical details and wanting to control my professional and personal world)—I find I am in daily conflict when trying to function as a surgeon.

I am a much softer person today, and I no longer am comfortable in the role of a surgeon. Though I have had much inner growth and made major changes in my focus over the past couple of years, I am still stuck with the baggage of my prior surgeon's personality. I have approached the limit of having further change in my current location, practice, and environment because of my inability to step away from my prior expectations and the "old" me.

This is really the crux of the dilemma. Do I want to totally change careers and perhaps go into counseling or hospice work, or would I still be happy being a surgeon if I were in another location where I could shed my prior baggage and function as I would now like to?

I am currently volunteering one day every other week for hospice. I spend two weeks a year doing volunteer surgery in Haiti. I like this type of work.

One option is working in hospice full-time, probably for some salary. A part-time position [in surgery] would probably be ideal, but they're hard to find. Another option is going back to school and getting a degree in counseling—perhaps with a focus on the suffering associated with dying and sick patients.

We proceeded with career consultation sessions (conducted by phone) in which we explored his options and dilemmas in greater depth. In addition, I coached Dr G on how to use the Internet to explore specific educational and career opportunities.

It opened a whole new world to him.

August 1998

Wow, am I overwhelmed! I guess that's good. My most exciting new thought of the day is that I became aware one can take courses for a certificate in gerontology at

University of South Florida in Tampa, which has one of the biggest gerontology departments in the country. And you can do it without having to go for a formal master's degree.

They have a wonderful course selection, including Death and Dying, and the opportunity to take counseling courses and then have supervision at local hospices. I spoke with the department chair, who was very helpful. I have a meeting with him in a couple of weeks. But as of now I am going to sign up for a graduate course on Death and Dying in the fall.

This avenue might give me an opportunity to get some formal training, as well as learn counseling skills in a more flexible way. If I decide to stay at our local hospice, I could get on-the-job medical training while taking courses. I'm also in the process of checking out some hospice meetings, as well as palliative care meetings. For me to ultimately get a job at a hospice, I certainly need more training and credentials.

In a short time I have become much more savvy at searching the Web. It's just very frustrating being in limbo without a definitive goal or plan.

Mid-August 1998

My current focus has been on hospice. I have found many courses, seminars, etc, which interest me and that I can use for continuing research and education. I have a tentative commitment that I can work at our local hospice in January.

I am registered at University of South Florida to take a Death and Dying course later this month. Perhaps I'm on my way to a certificate in gerontology with an emphasis on counseling. My current thoughts are to work at my local hospice for a year or so, get on-the-job training in the necessary primary care areas, and learn about [the workings of] hospice.

I have subscribed to Audio Digest family practice tapes to help educate me about general medical problems. I am joining the American Academy of Hospice and Palliative Medicine, which also serves as a credentialing board. Maybe if I become learned enough, I can ultimately get certified.

I sense that there are very few physicians with a commitment to hospice care and think this is a wide-open area for finding full- or part-time work. My current plan is to learn as much as I can, both on the job and with formal courses, and try to get credentialed.

Then, in a perfect world, I would get a job as a medical director in a hospice. I also found some hospice programs, retreats, and seminars with a Buddhist flavor. I think I can have the freedom to explore and practice compassion any way I want; so I feel the flexibility is there.

My biggest stumbling block is that every time I see an advertisement for a surgeon, I rethink my decision to stop doing surgery. It's hard to mentally give up and I'm still working through this. I think I have to grieve the loss of my identification as a surgeon and that's going to take some time.

October 1998

Just a brief follow-up. I am officially retiring from surgical practice and am going to be working full-time at our local hospice beginning in January. It really feels right and I'm very excited. I'm currently in the middle of my Death and Dying course at the University of Southern Florida.

I just came back from a four-day course at Duke, entitled Mind, Body and Spirituality in Medical Practice, and it was wonderful. I'm going to a three-day course for new hospice medical directors in St Louis in a couple of weeks. And finally, I'm enrolled in Joan Halifax's retreat/course, entitled Being with Dying, at Upaya in New Mexico in February. So I guess I'm on my way . . . .

Ongoing follow-up communication with Dr G confirms his continued satisfaction with his new professional identity.

References

Beckhard R, Pritchard W. *Changing the Essence: The Art of Creating and Leading Fundamental Change in Organizations.* San Francisco, Calif: Jossey-Bass Publishers; 1992.

Jaworski J. *Synchronicity: The Inner Path of Leadership.* San Francisco, Calif: Berrett-Koehler Publishers; 1996.

Klerman G. The joys and vicissitudes of life as a clinician-executive. In: Hirschowitz RG, Levy B, eds. *The Changing Mental Health Scene.* New York, NY: Spectrum Publications Inc; 1976:296-301.

Linney BJ. *Hope for the Future: A Career Development Guide for Physician Executives.* Tampa, Fla: American College of Physician Executives; 1996.

Pearson R, Haid, RL. The changing landscape of career development in medicine. *Career Plann and Dev J 14.* 1998;No. 1.

Raelin JA. *The Salaried Professional: How to Make the Most of Your Career.* New York, NY: Praeger Publishers; 1984.

Senge PM. *The Fifth Discipline: The Art & Practice of The Learning Organization.* New York, NY: Bantam Doubleday Dell Publishing Group Inc; 1990.

Tan JS. *Gender Issues in the Workplace: A Guide for Physician Executives.* Tampa, Fla: American College of Physician Executives; 1991.

Chapter 3

Professional versus Career Development

The American medical profession really doesn't have a framework, not to mention a language or lexicon, which it can easily and effectively use to discuss *career* development for physicians. It is possible, however, to discuss *professional* development. Indeed, professional development represents one of the cornerstones of modern American medicine. From the beginning, physicians are taught the importance of ongoing continuing medical education (CME) as a way to maintain clinical skills, stay abreast of the latest technical developments within their specialty, and often as documentation for license renewal.

But *career* development is not the same as *professional* development. Career paths are not defined simply by one's profession, but also by the roles and settings within which one applies his or her professional skills. For example, an orthopedist may practice clinically in a variety of settings, be an expert witness in malpractice trials, teach in an academic medical center, or work in product development or sales for a medical device company. It is the *range* and *sequence* of roles and employment settings that define one's *career path*.

Traditional medical education and training—both early in a physician's career and later in CME activities—focuses almost exclusively on professional development. Unfortunately, medical education at all stages fails to make physicians aware of the dramatic increase in recent years of employment options within virtually all specialties. This information gap compromises proactive and successful management of our careers.

▶ Professional Development

Professional development focuses on continually refining a narrowly defined area of expertise. It requires staying abreast of the latest research findings, as well as emerging technologies, in your specialty. Even within a single specialty, these challenges can be daunting. Although it always has been important to stay current in one's specialty, the pressures are even greater today. They may be fueled by "consumer" trends affecting the industry—the result of more and more medical topics covered both on the Internet and in the media. As the dizzying pace of new information increases in virtually every medical specialization, the pressure on physicians intensifies.

In addition, there is an increasing sense among physicians that we are too often ineffective in our professional roles. Donald Schön provides an eloquent discussion of the contention that professional knowledge (within medicine, as well as other professions) "... is mismatched to the changing character of the situations of practice—the complexity, uncertainty, instability, uniqueness and value conflicts which are increasingly perceived as central to the world of professional practice [today]." [1]

For some, this sense of ineffectiveness results from the feeling that traditional medicine has little to offer those patients whose symptoms are not relieved by this approach. Fortunately, these days physicians interested in complementary medicine can find CME programs that are venturing into these areas.

Another challenge for physicians today is to apply what they learned in their traditional medical training to practice in the "real" world. During their training, physicians are taught that performance excellence means leaving no stone unturned with patient care. But in today's managed care environment, the very behavior that elicited praise during education and training may well single you out as a "poor performer" in practice. It may even lead to reduced compensation or, worst case, dismissal from a group or managed care panel.

As eminent engineer and educator Harvey Brooks argues, the professions (including medicine) are now confronted with an "unprecedented requirement for adaptability." Although his point was made years ago, this astute observation remains timely for physicians in the current health care industry:

> *The dilemma of the professional today lies in the fact that both ends of the gap he is expected to bridge with his profession are changing so rapidly: the body of knowledge that he must use and the expectations of the society that he must serve. Both these changes have their origin in the same common factor—technological change. . . .*
>
> *The problem cannot be usefully phrased in terms of too much technology. Rather it is whether we can generate technological change fast enough to meet the expectations and demands that technology itself has generated. . . . This places on the professional a requirement for adaptability that is unprecedented.* [2]

---

[1] Schön DA. *The Reflective Practitioner: How Professionals Think in Action.* New York, NY: Basic Books Inc; 1983:14.

[2] Brooks H. The dilemmas of engineering education. *IEEE Spectrum.* February 1967:15.

◤ Career Development

To apply in a timely fashion for residency training, we physicians must make a key decision in our third or fourth year of medical school—which clinical specialty area to focus on. For many, this decision is made with little to no real information about the track we select. However, the fear of being too late in the application process outweighs our desire to learn more fully about available options.

Once the decision is made and we enter our residencies, we in effect put blinders on to block out anything that might distract us from achieving a critical level of mastery in our chosen specialty. Furthermore, once we commit to a specialty and to moving forward in this track, it is difficult to change to another track. This typically requires starting again at the beginning, rather than simply making an equivalent lateral move. This type of change, in addition to being psychologically difficult, often requires substantially more time, energy, and money, making it difficult logistically.

Strategic career development, on the other hand, proceeds most successfully when blinders are removed. Two important sources of information underlie successful career planning:

▼ Self-insight into what values, objectives, and goals are best aligned with career satisfaction

▼ Knowledge of the world around one's training, thus allowing for exploration of possible work settings and roles within which one's skills can be applied

Both of these items are typically neglected in traditional medical training programs. In fact, self-denial is essential for survival during these difficult years. It is critical for interns and residents to perform at high cognitive levels without eating or sleeping for prolonged periods of time, and this demands a certain level of self-denial. This state of self-denial occurs at the same time they need to exercise self-insight to select a specialty track that's "right" for them.

These two states of mind are often in conflict and lead to great confusion for many at this stressful and important stage of career development.

◤ Case Study

Dr Smith is a second-year surgical resident and is miserable.

I think I made a mistake going into surgery. I really had no idea what I wanted to go into. But it was time to apply for the match, so I had to make a decision. I had really admired my attending in surgery. He was so charismatic and smart, and he gave me such nice feedback. So I thought I would give that a try.

Now I realize I was trying to please him and, with the lack of any sense of what I really wanted to do, that was the only cue I had to follow. I will never be able to have the lifestyle I want as a surgeon. I don't really even like being in the OR that much, especially in comparison to how much my peers love being there.

The good news, though, is that making a career change, although not psychologically or logistically easy, is often done. Many physicians change their specialty, their organizational affiliation, and even their profession at some—or even several—points in their career.

There are many reasons why a physician may decide to make a career change. Reasons cited by approximately 750 physicians who have visited the Web site of MD IntelliNet (formerly MD CareerNet) [http://www.mdcareer.net] in search of career transition options include:

Actively plan and manage the next stage of my career	55%
Improve work-life balance	48%
Increase financial earning power	47%
Seek more opportunity for creativity	45%
Increase general quality of daily work life	41%
Reduce stress	39%
Incorporate greater intellectual challenge into my daily work	37%
Enhance my ability to make a difference in the world	34%
Add more variety to my work	33%
Address concerns about job security	29%
Work more as part of a collaborative team	24%
Adapt work to better accommodate personal/family phase of life situation	24%
Develop greater efficiency in my practice environment	14%
Plan a sabbatical	5%
Other	6%

◆ Career Transitions: Reactive vs Active

Career transitions may occur reactively—in response to newly defined needs that have been imposed upon an individual (eg, loss of medical license due to a disciplinary problem, recent onset of a debilitating health problem, or loss of job due to organizational downsizing). Yet ideally, the transition occurs as part of an *active* career plan (eg, arranging a job-sharing situation in anticipation of a new baby). An increasingly popular trend is for physicians to take an active role in their career direction through *diversification*. In other words, they add new dimensions to their current work without necessarily making a major transition.

Diversification can be a very effective way of increasing your marketability for future job searches. It also may enhance current personal and job satisfaction. If you're wondering what exactly you could do to diversify your career, here are four examples:

▼ Pediatrician in part-time clinical practice who consults with a health care software company

▼ Primary care physician who provides utilization review consultations for her managed care employer

▼ Director of clinical pharmacology in a major pharmaceutical company who contributes a regular column to an investment banking newsletter about biotechnology

▼ Family medicine physician who volunteers for one month each year in third world health care clinics

Individuals who work for large health care systems may have opportunities to diversify their professional experience by getting involved with any number of activities sponsored by their employer, even if it's on a volunteer basis. For example, interested physicians may become involved in technology assessment or drug formulary committees, or they might find a way to participate in an ongoing clinical trial. Such experiences can provide you with valuable perspectives, new skills, and the opportunity to meet people outside your profession—many of whom have the potential to help you in your quest for a more meaningful career.

Some within the medical profession with more traditional views feel that career diversification should be discouraged. They believe anything that dilutes your energy and focus might compromise your ability to be the best you can be in your primary clinical specialty. On the other hand, an increasing number of nontraditionalists have such a strong desire to broaden their skill sets and powers of influence that their views are moving quickly from the "radical fringe" to mainstream.

No matter which side you fall on, it is hard to disagree that career diversification can be a viable means of ensuring one's marketability within a rapidly changing industry. Whether becoming disabled due to a health problem or being laid off due to downsizing, physicians who have followed a traditional career path may well be at a disadvantage in finding alternative employment.

In addition, physicians in the current industry are clearly at greater risk of burnout as productivity demands escalate and their jobs more and more resemble assembly-line work. Adding variety to one's daily work can go a long way toward reducing burnout. Although the traditional model of professional development may still fit the needs and desires of some physicians, for a growing number this is no longer the case.

The nontraditionalist may only be seeking a broader range of experiences and skills as a physician. Still others may feel that their number one priority is career flexibility in anticipation of lifestyle issues. Whatever the rationale, it's crucial that physicians feel they can shape their careers to meet the demands of today's marketplace.

In Chapter 4 we will explore several career patterns that individuals may choose to pursue.

◭ Need for Flexible Work Arrangements

Although much of the focus in this book is on career diversification and transitions, it is important to acknowledge one other highly relevant set of issues strategic to career management: More and more physicians are interested in improving their work-life balance, and many do not want to leave clinical medicine in order to do it.

Unfortunately, arranging for part-time clinical work can be extremely difficult, if not impossible. By their very nature, some specialties cannot be easily practiced on a part-time basis (eg, cardiothoracic surgery). Furthermore, in some cases remaining credentialed and on the list of preferred providers of insurance or managed care organizations requires that a certain number of technical specialty procedures be performed annually by the physician. The sheer magnitude of this number in many cases essentially precludes the possibility of part-time practice.

In addition, part-time practice is discouraged in subtle ways within employer organizations and the profession itself. For example, part-timers talk quietly of feeling exploited (half-time is actually three-quarters time in terms of responsibilities and on-call duties, but not pay).

Finally, there is little open discussion about models for flexible work, such as job-sharing, much less sanctioned channels by which those interested in job-sharing can find each other. As we move into the 21st century, it is hoped there will be a growing recognition within the profession, as well as in health care organizations, that it is a sign of health that an increasing number of physicians see work-life balance as a priority.

Workaholism has long been recognized as a pathological trait within the medical profession. It has taken its toll on many physicians, their families, health care organizations, and patients. However, it is not enough for individual physicians to make a personal decision to reduce their work hours. We now need to legitimize flexible and part-time work schedules for physicians by institutionalizing them through practical definitions, structure, and support within organizational settings and credentialing systems.

References

Hackman JR, Oldham GR. *Work Redesign.* Reading, Mass: Addison-Wesley Publishing Company; 1980.

Heckscher C. *White Collar Blues.* New York, NY: HarperCollins Publishers Inc; 1995.

Levine S. Some problematic aspects of medicine's changing status. In: Hafferty FW, McKinley JB, eds. *The Changing Medical Profession: An International Perspective.* New York, NY: Oxford University Press; 1993.

Nash DB. *Future Practice Alternatives in Medicine.* New York, NY: Igaku-Shoin; 1993.

Schön, DA. *The Reflective Practitioner: How Professionals Think in Action.* New York, NY: Basic Books Inc; 1983.

Chapter 4

Four Career Concepts

◆ On Being a Physician: By Design or by Default?

If asked when and why they decided to become a physician, a surprising number respond that they never really planned it. Rather it seemed to just "happen." Or as one of my clients quipped, "It was decided for me in utero."

Indeed, some enter medicine as a means of pleasing some authority figure or role model, such as their parents. Many physicians are ultimately satisfied with their career choice, no matter how they came to it. But for others, the outcome is less than satisfying.

Historically, the choice to become a physician also has been influenced by many social forces—status, respect, and security. So for many families, a medical degree represents the ultimate in success. If this opportunity was beyond the reach of the preceding generation, they may view it for their progeny as a "prize" worth attaining at any cost.

These dynamics lead many to pursue medical school as a *means to an image* rather than a *line of work*. For many of these individuals, it soon becomes clear that the daily realities of being a physician are at odds with the image being pursued.

Early in one's training, though, it is difficult to know if that growing dissatisfaction and disillusionment will subside as one progresses into residency and then into posttraining practice. To further complicate any change of heart, the sheer investment of time, finances, and energy in the training process creates a real or perceived curtailing of options. As a result, many young physicians remain in clinical medicine, only to have their early doubts confirmed in practice.

The key to career satisfaction is to actively shape your career path. Each career decision should be guided by an understanding of all your options and whether they align with your own objectives.

◗ The Career Concepts Model

What follows is an introduction to *Career Concepts*, a conceptual framework defined by Kenneth R. Brousseau, PhD, and Michael J. Driver, PhD.[1] This model emerged from 25 years of meticulous research in industrial psychology. Its subjects were high-level technical professionals, managers, and executives. However, as business has reshaped the lives of those working in health care, the value of the Career Concepts model has become applicable to physicians as well.

Physicians who effectively manage their careers not only achieve greater *personal* satisfaction but also contribute more to organizational success. Thus, this model is increasingly being used as a resource by individual physicians, as well as by the managers, human resource personnel, and consultants who work with them.

Career Concepts describe different types of careers. Physicians often differ from one another in the way they think about careers and in the types of careers they believe are most desirable. Most of these differences concern:

▼ the stability of one's profession, specialty, and practice setting;

▼ vertical (up a "ladder") vs horizontal/lateral career moves; and

▼ the duration of one's stay in a particular field.

Career Concepts address these issues in describing four fundamentally different types of careers.

◗ Four Basic Career Concepts

Research indicates that four fundamental career concepts depict how different individuals view the ideal career. These concepts are:

> Linear
>
> Expert
>
> Spiral
>
> Transitory

Each of these concepts is described in detail, followed by descriptions of their various hybrids. Within these four basic concepts can be found most possible career patterns.

---

[1] Brousseau KR, Driver MJ. Enhancing informed choice: a career-concepts approach to career advisement. *Selections.* Spring 1994:24-31.

Linear Career Concept

The linear view revolves around how high one rises in a hierarchy. Under this definition, success is based on increasing levels of responsibility, authority, status, and reward. In the linear view, the worst of all fates is to be "stalled" in one's career. In other words, career stagnation is the kiss of death.

Many who subscribe to the linear career concept as their personal model of success view upward mobility as the only acceptable path. They often find it difficult to imagine how anyone could define success differently.

For physicians, upward career movement typically involves rising to higher and higher levels in the management hierarchy of their organization. Management roles for physicians, in general, remain limited to clinical staff management. It is rare for the authority of physician managers to be extended beyond the clinical to the *operational* side of an organization.

Thus, in most cases, physician management roles are not "line" management roles but remain restricted to "functional" management positions. It is also generally the case today that physicians seeking more managerial authority must independently seek additional training in business administration or management.

◤ Case Study

Linear Career Concept

Mark Frankel, MD, is currently in his third year of a pediatrics residency and, by all accounts, has performed extremely well. In addition to receiving honors in all of his major clinical rotations, he has won several research awards from pharmaceutical companies for clinical research done during his training.

He has been accepted in one of the country's top hematology/oncology fellowship programs following his residency.

Despite this stellar track record, Dr Frankel feels unsettled about his career. He describes how difficult it is for him to watch his nonphysician friends and colleagues make substantially more money than he does. He is increasingly frustrated that this will continue at least until he completes his fellowship.

He is also envious when he sees his friends receive promotions in their jobs, resulting in greater status and compensation, whereas he faces the prospect of first-year fellow, which sentences him yet again to being "low man on the totem pole."

Even when he imagines proceeding with his fellowship, it is hard for him to envision career satisfaction. What opportunities will there be for him to distinguish himself (ie, advance his career) once he enters practice?

Simply having a successful practice doesn't seem enough to him. He is interested in redirecting his career out of clinical medicine, either into investment banking or a pharmaceutical company. In these settings he sees himself best suited as an executive.

Expert Career Concept

From a historical point of view, the expert career concept has perhaps been around the longest. It is consistent with the philosophy behind the guild structure of occupations that originated in Europe during the Middle Ages and that still largely exists within medicine.

Under this system, a vocational ladder—much like the professional development of physicians—has three key rungs: apprentice ("see one"), journeyman ("do one"), and master ("teach one"). Ultimate career success means mastering the most difficult and esoteric aspects of one's discipline. The expert view of success differs sharply from the linear view. From the perspective of the expert, success results from finding one's "calling" and becoming more and more skilled in that.

Advancement in this model depends on deepening one's level of *technical expertise*—not on how many people one supervises, the size of one's office, or the size of one's paycheck. Despite the emphasis so many organizations place on the linear concept of moving up the ranks (where managers often do less "hands-on" work with each promotion), the expert concept represents legitimacy in many professional circles. Physicians who view success in expert terms may have real reservations about a linear ladder that may distance them from their specialized knowledge.

Case Study

Expert Career Concept

John Jasper, MD, a 55-year-old cardiothoracic surgeon, just turned down an offer to become chief of staff in a teaching hospital affiliated with a major academic center. He is currently Chief of Surgery there and accepted this role only because his mentor formerly held the position and strongly encouraged him to be his replacement when he retired.

Dr Jasper hates committee meetings, managing people, and dealing with bureaucracy. These time-consuming and often exasperating activities only serve to keep him from what he enjoys most: surgery.

He originally chose a career in academic medicine because it allowed him access to clinical research facilities, to the latest technology, and to the most challenging clinical cases. Also, each promotion ensured greater job security.

And when he first made this career choice, surgeons in academia operated on patients, while administrators operated hospital business. But of late, more and more administrative activities are focusing on departmental and hospital changes resulting from a recent merger. Dr Jasper is increasingly frustrated that so much of his time and energy are consumed by administrative matters.

Consequently, although he has always loved his surgical career, he is considering retirement within the next few years—much sooner than ever expected.

Spiral Career Concept

Compared to linear and expert definitions of success, the spiral career concept is a much less traditional mind-set, although it probably has been around "unofficially" for some time.

From the spiral perspective, success means a progressive *broadening* of one's knowledge, skills, and expertise over time. As a pattern of movement, the spiral career usually begins with a particular specialty, then moves periodically into new fields and types of work. The average move occurs every 5 to 10 years.

This spiral movement may offer little or no career promotion. Instead, the key consideration is the new learning that comes from a different type of work. Yet rather than being random, the moves have a definite pattern. Each new field of work:

▼ requires the use of previously acquired skills or knowledge and

▼ opens the door to opportunities to develop new knowledge and skills.

Thus, the term *spiral* connotes a career pattern that spirals outward from some central core set of competencies. Even though the spiral concept has not thus far been formally recognized in the career literature, it does accurately describe many people—physicians included—who are seen as successful for their breadth of experience, versatility, and range of skills. The term *self-actualization* also captures important aspects of the spiral career by stressing full achievement of one's potential.

Many physicians who fit the spiral model may not pursue it because they don't even know that it exists. When the concept is introduced to them, recognition often comes in a flash: "That's me! That's what I really want!" Other spiral types know very well what they are trying to do with their careers, although they may not feel comfortable talking about it to those who see success in only linear or expert terms.

But as the spiral concept becomes a more legitimate and desirable way of thinking about career success, many people have come forward who otherwise might have remained "closet-spirals." Often these individuals have felt held captive by more traditional career tracks.

◤ Case Study

Spiral Career Concept

Sally Chang, MD, a 45-year-old internist, is presently doing a special fellowship on health care policy analysis at Harvard University's Kennedy School of Government. This is not the first time since completing her medical residency she has taken leave from patient care to obtain more academic training—namely a master's in public health, then a master's in business administration, and now the policy fellowship.

Dr Chang says she's back in school out of a desire to expand her range of professional skills. From her perspective as a clinician, she has observed a number of problems within the health care system—lack of attention to and resources for prevention; poor management of limited health care resources; and ineffective, poorly conceptualized health care policies that compromise care delivery.

By broadening her skills and expertise, she hopes to shift her focus from direct patient care to activities that allow her to improve the health care system overall, within her organization, as well as on the state and national levels.

She also notes that one of her great professional pleasures, particularly as she moves forward in her own career development, is being a mentor to younger women physicians.

Transitory Career Concept

This fourth concept is even less traditional than the spiral concept— especially for physicians. A transitory career involves patterns of movement best described as "consistent inconsistency."

From the transitory perspective, the ideal career consists of a fascinating smorgasbord of experiences. People who pursue transitory careers change jobs or type of work an average of every two to four years. Unlike the spiral career concept, which involves an orderly progression of related work experiences, the transitory pattern is most clearly defined when a person moves from one type of work to another that is totally different. The more distinct the difference, the better and brighter the opportunity when viewed from the transitory perspective.

It can be quite challenging for true transitory physicians to avoid feeling frustrated and restless within a traditional medical career. They may cope with their need for frequent change by taking time off during medical school and residency or by choosing a clinical specialty with "built-in" variety and movement (eg, emergency medicine). Ultimately, they may use their medical training and credentials as a platform for moving into sectors outside of clinical medicine rather than remaining in clinical practice for an extended period of time. Interestingly, many people whose careers clearly show the transitory pattern believe that they don't really have a career and they "really should figure out what I want to do when I grow up!"

A transitory physician is likely to feel he or she "just doesn't fit in" with colleagues or the system. What this reflects is that they work best "outside the box" of a traditionally defined medical career. Yet intellectually (though not emotionally or motivationally) they've accepted these traditional definitions.

The transitory concept, though, *does represent a real and legitimate approach to a career.* It has definite characteristics: many diverse experiences, frequent movement, and little or no emphasis on upward movement. Most important, it captures the type of career many people want when they realistically face their own needs and motives, without the ever-present, outside interference of "social programming." For the unconflicted and confirmed transitory, a career can be an endless adventure.

◢ Case Study

Transitory Career Concept

Beth Kelly, MD, found medical school boring. The least boring clinical rotation was in the emergency room, where she enjoyed the fast pace, the unpredictability, and the variety of each shift. She decided to volunteer for a variety of electives related to emergency medicine, including:

▼ working at a crisis center on a remote Indian reservation;

▼ doing shifts in the field with EMS workers;

▼ participating in a major clinical trial in the department; and

▼ participating in a focus group of clinicians regarding a support software system for the department.

After completing her residency in emergency medicine, she obtained a part-time position in the department. Alongside her clinical work, she maintained an independent consulting practice in the medical device and information technology industries. She advised her clients on marketing and business development, in particular, activities that targeted emergency departments. Within her department, she was known as a "change agent" and innovator of new projects and programs.

Three years after assuming her job in the emergency department, she decided it was time for a change. She was soon hired as medical director of a multimedia medical education company.

Career Concepts and Career Motives

How is it that people differ so dramatically in the career experiences they want? For the transitory person, an expert career would be akin to a life of bondage. Yet for the expert person, a transitory career would be a life of superficiality, possibly even insanity.

In looking at people who seem to be most clear about the career pattern they want, certain underlying motives are apparent. Each career pattern has its own set of rewards that distinguishes it from the other career patterns. This is what we see when we look at the motives of people who subscribe to different career concepts.

Linear Motives

One of the most noteworthy features of those most committed to the linear concept is that they want a lot of different rewards in their careers. That said, the motive most strongly linked to the linear career is power. The power motive usually is followed by the achievement motive. In short, linear people want to be "movers and shakers." In today's health care organizations, the best way to do this is to climb the ladder to positions of ever-greater influence and authority.

Expert Motives

Most notable about the expert type is that they want to become as proficient in their work as possible. In most cases, they also want to be recognized by others for their expertise. But for many, the most essential motive is the self-knowledge that they excel in their chosen fields.

Security often comes second. The stronger the commitment to the expert career, the more likely these physicians do *not* want novelty, job mobility, or power over people. They want stable and predictable situations in which they are free to develop and exercise their skills. If they have this, they are often the most satisfied people in the organization.

Spiral Motives

Spiral-minded people are like their linear counterparts in that they usually want many things. However, the motive that usually gets the highest rating is personal growth. They want to develop substantial skills in a variety of fields over time.

Following the motive for personal growth are several others that are in close competition with each other. These include:

▼ creativity, or the desire to be involved in new developments and trailblazing efforts, and

▼ nurturance, as reflected in helping others grow and develop; for this reason, spiral types often make excellent mentors.

Transitory Motives

The prime motive of people pursuing transitory careers is variety or novelty. Also high on their lists are independence and involvement with people.

What this says is that transitories are strongly motivated to get involved in new projects or enterprises with other people, particularly in situations where they are free to exercise their own judgment without the constraints of bureaucracy. They also tend to enjoy and be very adept at "networking," or meeting different types of people. Not surprisingly, many transitory physicians are entrepreneurs or independent consultants at some point in their careers.

▷ Special Challenges for Each Career Concept

Just as each career concept has its own set of potential rewards, each also has its own challenges, which one should be aware of when planning a career. The linear career physician, for example, actually has more potential growth opportunities now than ever before in the health care industry. As the clinical services sector has consolidated, a significant need has arisen for well-qualified physicians to assume general management positions. However, the linear career type may find his or her aspirations to climb the corporate ladder frustrated by a glass ceiling imposed by executives who tend to view physicians as not being "business people." (This topic will be discussed in greater depth in Chapter 8.)

The challenge of the expert career is to avoid the threat of obsolescence because of an increasing volume of information and the pace of new research and technology.

It is often difficult for mid- to late-career experts to compete with their younger counterparts, who have been trained in the latest technical developments. Another challenge for the physician expert results from the massive restructuring of health care organizations, which may disrupt his or her need for stability and security.

Physicians as a group are well known within organizations to be highly resistant to change. Typically, those who demonstrate this tendency the most are the experts. The spiral and transitory physicians are less threatened by the organizational changes taking place in health care today. In general, these types benefit from restructuring that reduces hierarchy and bureaucracy because this may eliminate barriers to potential lateral movement.

Yet despite such changes, most organizational policies remain more supportive of linear or expert careers. Physicians pursuing a spiral career path will generally find that they need to be proactive about identifying, and often creating, lateral opportunities.

The general phenomenon all physicians face of being pigeonholed is an even greater challenge for transitories. Larger and more bureaucratic organizations, in particular, tend to typecast according to training and background. In many places, a resume that indicates a transitory career pattern is interpreted as "flaky" or unreliable, even though these same organizations may need people who are willing to go anywhere, anytime, to tackle a new project or solve an urgent problem.

The greatest challenge facing all of us physicians, regardless of career concept, is to plan and organize our careers to support the central motives that are important to us as individuals. This is why self-insight is a powerful and essential tool in career planning. Without it, the prospect of enjoying a rewarding career is primarily a matter of luck.

◆ Beyond Primary Concepts: Hybrid Career Concept Patterns

Many people have one strong career concept and a second concept that is nearly as strong. It is useful to look at these as "hybrids." These combined patterns provide the richest indicator of your ideal career pathway.

The six major hybrid patterns are described in detail in the following paragraphs. Research data correlate each pattern with a particular type of management career outside of the physician workforce. This makes it somewhat challenging to map these nonmedical career tracks to the professional world of physicians. However, once again drawing from MD IntelliNet's client archives, these hybrid patterns can be illustrated by individual cases, as noted in the following chart.

Hybrid Career Concepts

Hybrid Career Concept	Classic Nonphysician Career Track	Sample Physician Career Track
Linear/Expert Expert/Linear	Functional manager	Chief of surgery Medical director of dialysis center
Linear/Spiral Spiral/Linear	Generalist manager	Editor of major professional journal Chief information officer of HMO
Linear/Transitory Transitory/Linear	Independent business owner/manager	President of small, entrepreneurial practice group
Expert/Spiral Spiral/Expert	General consultant	Physician with specialty- specific role in management consulting firm
Expert/Transitory Transitory/Expert	Independent consultant	ER physician, independent consultant to device/IT industries
Spiral/Transitory Transitory/Spiral	Entrepreneur/ Intrapreneur	Internist who successfully starts up and sells two medical software companies

Linear/Expert Hybrid
Expert/Linear Hybrid

The linear-expert hybrid fits best on a track that involves climbing a career ladder in one's field, using demonstrated technical competence as the basis for advancement. This is generally thought of as the functional manager career track. For nonphysicians, this traditionally has been the most common and surest route to the highest-level positions.

For physicians, however, this is generally not the case. As noted earlier, their authority tends to remain limited to the clinical side of organizations and rarely extends into the operations side, where business executives are usually positioned. That said, physicians may well rise to a respected position high on the functional management ladder.

In selecting the functional manager track, it is important to choose an organization where the area in which you plan to develop your expertise is highly valued. For example, if your specialty is Physical Medicine and Rehabilitation, your opportunity for advancement on the functional management ladder is likely much greater in a rehabilitation facility than in a general academic medical center.

Linear/Spiral Hybrid
Spiral/Linear Hybrid

The linear-spiral pattern fits best with the general manager career track that is becoming increasingly common outside of the medical profession. Instead of selecting senior managers whose backgrounds are limited to one function, many large organizations now rotate managers through a series of functions in different areas to develop well-rounded executives with a global perspective on the business.

Unfortunately, such lateral opportunities for physicians to expand their professional knowledge and skills within the context of the job are extremely rare. Instead, their career opportunities are often rigidly matched to what is perceived as a narrow range of skills and expertise.

There are, however, an increasing number of roles within the broader health care industry that can be highly satisfying for physicians oriented toward the spiral concept. The dramatic changes in the industry have created many new products and services that can benefit from a physician's valuable expertise. Generally it is up to the individual physician to be creative, resourceful, and active in finding such opportunities, which are often independent of their employer organization.

In striving to satisfy the linear component of one's career concept, again the individual physician must create his or her own management track. In some organizations, this may well define new territory for physician managers.

Linear/Transitory Hybrid
Transitory/Linear Hybrid

In the business world, the linear-transitory career pattern perhaps fits best with an independent business owner/manager of a small but growing company. These organizations are usually more flexible and can shift directions relatively easily. They also provide opportunity for rapid advancement.

A physician with a linear-transitory hybrid concept would likely find satisfaction as the entrepreneurial manager of a small clinical practice group, pursuing a range of opportunities in the evolving marketplace.

Expert/Spiral Hybrid Expert/Transitory Hybrid
Spiral/Expert Hybrid, Transitory/Expert Hybrid

Both of these hybrid patterns are a particularly good fit with a career in consulting. The difference between them lies in the type of consulting one does and for what type of organization.

The expert-spiral hybrid fits best with fairly complex consulting in highly specialized disciplines. An example would be a surgeon working with a management consulting firm that specializes in the development and management of ambulatory surgical care centers. Other desirable consulting activities could be helping to develop new medical software, assisting an organization in a new business strategy, or any other organizational innovation. For many physicians that fit the expert-spiral pattern, working in the clinical services sector will not provide the innovation and creativity important to their career satisfaction.

The expert-transitory hybrid suits independent consultants. Consulting projects are typically short, and the consultant may be called upon to perform a variety of services. Ideally, the expert-transitory consultant will have the opportunity to move rapidly from one project to another, while applying a basic set of expert skills and knowledge. Trouble-shooting and turnaround projects—such as redefining the marketing strategy for a new medical device or modifying the user interface of a specialized medical software product—fit the expert-transitory hybrid very well.

Spiral/Transitory Hybrid
Transitory/Spiral Hybrid

The spiral-transitory is the pattern of the pure entrepreneur, one who starts and sells one business after another. It also applies to the organizational intrapreneur, who is seen as a "spark plug" or "change agent" and is given wide berth to get new projects, products, or services underway. The key here is lots of variety, creative accomplishment, and independence from stultifying policies and procedures (eg, the traditional academic medical center).

Note: If you'd like to learn more about your career profile, an online *CareerView Assessment* tool is provided through my company at http://www.mdintellinet.com (click on Assessment Tools on the Home Page). There is an administrative charge for this service.

Reference

Brousseau KR, Driver MJ, Eneroth K, Larsson R. Career pandemonium: realigning organizations and individuals. *Acad Manage Executives 10.* 1996;No. 4:1-22.

Chapter 5

Career Diversification and Transitions

Career diversification differs from career transition in that a transition generally represents a complete change from your primary professional role into a new one. Career diversification usually occurs by taking on additional activities alongside of your primary professional role. Diversification enables you to add new skills and experiences to your work, while maintaining the security of your current job.

Career transitions are often executed by first establishing a "bridge" from one's current career path to the target path. Diversification activities can serve as that bridge, thus minimizing the risk involved in the transition. It is important to select your diversification activities strategically, with an eye toward your evolving interests and priorities for your next career stage.

Thus, diversification activities may be:

▼ additional tasks and/or responsibilities within your health care organization but outside of your core job description;

▼ designed to broaden your experiences, skills, and contacts in a part-time way, while remaining primarily anchored in direct patient care;

▼ focused on something that relates to your clinical specialty, although not necessarily involving direct patient care;

▼ often a volunteer activity, at least initially; or

▼ potentially, but not necessarily, a stepping-stone to a significant career transition.

All of the above represent a short-term investment of time, energy, and possibly money that may pay off in long-term control and greater personal and professional satisfaction. In addition, diversification activities often lie on a continuum with transitions, allowing one to "test the waters" in a new area of professional activity before making a major leap.

You may even try different diversification activities over time and, through these experiences and contacts, decide what you like in particular. You might then design a bridge that targets this type of work and thus make a methodical transition in that direction. Or you may decide to remain in direct patient care but use these diversification activities part-time for some variety in your work life.

⮚ Creating a Plan for Change

Many physicians, once they decide that they want a change, have a fantasy that the perfect opportunity will simply come to them. My experience is that such serendipity is very rare. When it does occur, it tends to happen to those physicians who already have industry experience. For instance, I am aware of situations involving a high-level physician executive who got a call from a recruiter in the insurance industry, or a well-known academic physician with well-publicized research experience who received a call from a pharmaceutical company.

For the sake of discussion, let's assume such an opportunity for change "dropped into your lap." What now? Experience has shown me that the time spent making a plan is time well spent. A plan need not be laborious or highly detailed, but it should be more than just saying to yourself, "I want a change."

Any plan should take the following into consideration.

Your Objectives. For example, do you want to increase your earning power in your current situation? Or do you seek a better work-life balance?

A Realistic Timeline. For instance, to make a move out of clinical medicine altogether, the ideal plan allows for a two- or three-year transition period.

What Direction You Wish to Go. Perhaps most challenging for many full-time clinicians is how to focus new activities so they lead in the right direction.

Your decision to make a change may be driven by external factors, or it may be driven by internal forces. But in guiding the direction of the process, ideally you should match your interests to emerging marketplace opportunities. (Chapter 7 provides an in-depth look at how to do the market research to identify these opportunities.)

This is a highly personalized process, which is precisely why someone else cannot create the plan for you. It's crucial that you yourself sift through the options, become informed about the market, and reflect on personal interests and priorities.

We will not focus in this chapter on plans that take a physician totally outside of health care. Before taking such a radical step, I believe disgruntled physicians should try to leverage their medical degrees if at all possible. They may be surprised to discover this can increase not only personal and professional satisfaction but market value as well.

◀ Case Study

Dr B: New Lease on Life

This Web site visitor found that working part-time in a new area of clinical medicine allowed him the flexibility to pursue another long-standing passion. He offers his story to encourage those who want to make a change but are afraid to take the steps to do so:

I'm 50 and a board-certified family doctor who left practice 2 years ago after 19 years. Our practice had been acquired by XXX Practice Management Company and mismanaged right into the ground.

Fortunately, I realized I was ready for a change. I did locum tenens work every other month for the first year and now work two 10-hour days a week in our hospital's workman's compensation clinic. Surprisingly, I had my second best [income] year ever last year—working half-time.

I love to work on houses. Over the last two years (after refinancing our house), we acquired 10 rental houses, which I've fixed up. All are rented at positive cash flow. We're in debt to the hilt, yet my stress level is the lowest since life before medical school.

◀ Defining Your Options

The most common reason physicians who want to make a career change get "stuck" is lack of knowledge about their options. Why is the range of options such an unknown for physicians? When physicians are in training, our ability to learn about nonacademic positions is usually hindered by the moat surrounding the Ivory Towers of academe. So any awareness of the commercial marketplace, where other options lie, is extremely limited.

> *Structures of which we are unaware hold us prisoner.*
> —Peter M. Senge, *The Fifth Discipline*

Once young physicians commit to a clinical specialty, their worldview becomes further narrowed by the intense training required for certification. Then the daily demands of clinical practice substantially limit how much time and energy they have to explore any nontraditional dimensions of health care that might greatly enrich their careers.

In mid- to late practice, physicians gradually become aware of how limited their professional lives have become. Yet by this time, they likely have developed a great deal of confidence and mastery in their specialty, even while wanting new kinds of professional opportunities. Many become frustrated by not knowing how to diversify.

Many of my physician clients go through an initial phase where they can't succinctly articulate what their interests are outside of their core specialty. They can only express a vague sense of what they want to do and in what general direction.

As noted earlier, the process of diversification usually takes active exploration (using the Internet, networking, information gathering, reading, etc). This exploration is essential to get you to the point where you can articulate your new direction or niche in one or two sentences, so that, as they say, if you were to find yourself on an elevator with someone of great influence, you could clearly convey your new target career before they exit at the next floor.

One of the advantages of networking (see Chapter 6) is that you pick up the lingo of other businesses and industries. The ability to speak to someone in their professional language is critical.

It cannot be overemphasized: Your *personal involvement* is required. No recruiter is going to be able to make these decisions for you. Becoming facile in your search can, in and of itself, give you a satisfying sense of mastery. Because growth and development never cease, the skills you develop are critical to ongoing career management.

◣ Career Guidance for the Medical Student or Resident

At this early point in your career, actively creating a special niche, alongside the requisite activities, can provide a strategic advantage that will benefit you not only during training but well into the future. For example, the right inquiries can help you determine what clinical trials may be underway and whether you can participate as a member of the investigative team. This allows interested students to see if they enjoy clinical research and introduces them to new colleagues, as well as pharmaceutical representatives. Such contacts may lead to future opportunities, either within academia, private practice, or the pharmaceutical industry. It is important to make such contacts early on. Once formal training is completed, it can be difficult or impossible to get involved in clinical trials at an entry level.

Another way to test the waters is through extracurricular activities. Medical students often have access to classes outside the confines of their medical education—at an affiliated school of public health, for example. There also may be clubs to join—if not within the medical school itself, then in related health care institutions (eg, a medical informatics club). Many such opportunities are free and build relationships outside the clinical training track.

Once you have defined your areas of interest, you might set up informational interviews with commercial health care enterprises in your local area (or the area you'd like to live in after graduation) to learn how they work with physicians. You also might arrange meetings with other physicians who work for such companies. You may see if you could volunteer for a period of time—something like a corporate internship. Such arrangements often lead to future consulting or employment opportunities.

How you plan your strategy will differ from individual to individual. The important thing is to take advantage of the range of formal and informal resources available to you while you are in medical training. Above all, be assertive about finding these contacts. They will not come to you. Yet once forged, they may become some of the most valuable and long-lasting ones of your career.

◢ Career Diversification Strategies for Physicians in Training

Physicians in training can use any of the following career diversification strategies.

▼ Create a nontraditional niche that you can build alongside your required curriculum.

▼ Identify and participate in diversified activities—either formally or informally— within your medical school, training hospital, or related institutions.

▼ Find professional associations to join, either local or national, that focus on issues relevant to your niche.

▼ Network with individuals and companies that share your interests and see if there are ways to collaborate.

▼ If possible, establish visibility in your niche through writing and speaking activities.

◣ Career Diversification Strategies for Mid-career Clinicians

A mid-career clinician can use several strategies in his or her career diversification. Some may want to pursue interests that naturally evolve from their ongoing clinical work (eg, integrative medicine or bioethics). Others may want to connect their current work with interests and skills that developed earlier in their careers (eg, parlay an undergraduate computer engineering degree with one's clinical experience in the arena of health care information technology).

How you go about creating such niches depends, in part, on what your goals are. Some may simply want to add new dimensions to their lives. Others may be more goal oriented (eg, create new revenue-generating activities). If the latter is the case, it is important that any new niche be marketplace driven. That is, know your industry trends so the niche can be defined in a way that maximizes its marketability.

As a clinician in practice today, one of the most challenging issues is how to establish the time and energy needed to pursue diversification activities. Ideally, one-half to one full day per week should be set aside for such activities. Whenever possible, this should be scheduled for the same time each week. Knowing that you have every Wednesday afternoon reserved for your new career goal can lend some structure to an otherwise highly unstructured process.

Once you have created the requisite space in your life, you are then ready to proceed:

▼ Select an area of general interest to explore for any potential expert niche that could be developed.

▼ Consider ways you might participate in related activities at affiliated clinical institutions or outside organizations. These may be with key individuals, groups, or committees.

▼ Find out what is happening in national and international associations that is related to your desired niche. Some may have local or regional affiliations. Attend an annual meeting and explore ways to collaborate with newfound contacts who share your interest.

▼ Read any and all mailings from associations you join for valuable perspectives on market trends, marketing strategies, and potential professional partners.

▼ Network with companies and organizations that may have an interest in you and your evolving expertise (the concept of networking is discussed in Chapter 6).

▼ Take an academic course in your new area of interest at a local graduate school. This is also a good way to network with people who can share their perspectives of the market as it relates to your niche.

▼ Create a Web site as a cost-effective marketing and distribution channel for your evolving activities.

▼ Make a new business card that defines the new you!

◢ Case Study

Dr Z: Finding the Right Fit

This was actually a fairly complicated case that took a number of years to unfold. It was one where the tool for organizing issues into the personal/professional/

organizational spheres was quite useful in sorting out priorities. Dr Z's tenacious efforts to find professional satisfaction were inspiring to observe.

When Dr Z first came to see me, she was so miserable it was difficult to sort out her problems. We initially decided her working style was incompatible with that of her employer (an HMO). She tried a different practice setting, and the fit was much better. She was happier for several years, but then underlying discontent with her role as a primary care physician began to resurface.

After further sessions, we decided she would likely never find a better fit than what she currently had in her organizational setting. So it was probably time to address the possibility of a less than good fit between Dr Z and direct patient care.

Dr Z was 38 and worked in a small group practice affiliated with a community teaching hospital. This was her second practice setting in the past eight years. She had become convinced she was never going to love medicine again, no matter what the setting.

Early in her career she was involved in bench research, but she did not want to return to that. She had been exploring many sources of information trying to discover her career options. She began to use the Internet as part of her search and realized she enjoyed doing research that way. I found her a part-time, entry-level position in a start-up health care Internet company near her home.

Although she did this work on a volunteer basis, she decided it would be time and energy well spent. It gave her an opportunity to learn more about the Internet, as well as what it is like to work in an entrepreneurial start-up environment.

After four months there, she decided she definitely wanted to leave clinical practice and develop skills in computer programming. Two months later she began taking computer programming courses part-time while continuing her volunteer work at the Internet company. When we last spoke, this company was considering her for hire. She also was exploring other job openings in the computer industry, both within and outside of health care.

In reflecting on her unhappiness in her career as a practicing clinician, Dr Z now sees clearly that she was simply not cut out to be a physician. Although she is anxious to find stable employment in her new career, she is comfortable—at least for now—that computer programming feels right.

◗ Planning Your Retirement

For many physicians, the expertise they develop throughout their career becomes the primary focus of their activities after retiring from clinical practice. For those who want to remain professionally active during retirement, having a foundation already built for this focus can make the transition more orderly, less disorienting, and actually quite pleasant.

Career Diversification Strategies for Retirement

As retirement draws near, develop contacts in the geographic area where you plan to settle who share your interests and will form a new community of colleagues and associates. Participate in their local activities, even in small ways from a distance, before relocating.

Identify commercial institutions in that geographic area that may be interested in hiring you as a consultant or member of an advisory board. Schedule introductory meetings with them. Identify organizations that might benefit from your area of expertise. See if you can structure a role for yourself as a volunteer within their activities.

◢ Sample Career Diversification Activities

The range of possible career diversification activities you can identify or create for yourself is truly limitless. Here is a list—not complete by any means—of some things you can do to begin to diversify. This list is generated from what my clients have done on a part-time basis as they gradually cut back their full-time clinical practice. They chose these activities for many reasons: for the sake of variety, to open new doors, to explore a personal passion, etc.

▼ Assume part-time medical directorship of a skilled nursing facility.

▼ Assume part-time medical directorship at a prison facility.

▼ Conduct independent medical evaluations for workers' compensation, disability, malpractice, utilization review, and quality assurance.

▼ Become a consultant to a health care investment banking firm—helping them evaluate potential investment opportunities.

▼ Become a consultant to a pharmaceutical market research firm.

▼ Take mediation training with subsequent involvement in arbitration within insurance companies.

▼ Become a consultant to a medical software company, providing them with medical expertise for their content development.

▼ Get involved in multilevel marketing of botanical supplements.

▼ Join a speakers bureau for pharmaceutical companies.

▼ Develop multimedia educational materials for pharmaceutical companies.

▼ Recruit appropriate patients from your practice into clinical trials.

▼ Establish your practice as an investigative site and contract with site management organizations to do clinical trials.

▼ Volunteer to participate in one of the following types of committees in your hospital or managed care organization:

Pharmacy and therapeutics
Technology assessment
Institutional review board
Clinical trials safety
Continuing education
Patient education
Patient advocacy
Physician health/well-being
Medical staff credentials
Bioethics

▼ Participate in survey teams that provide accreditation to hospitals and managed care organizations.

▼ Volunteer to work part-time with your state board of registration in medicine.

▼ Join an advisory board of a start-up company or nonprofit organization.

▼ Help your department or organization develop its Web site and patient education materials.

▼ Join the editorial advisory board of a professional or lay publication.

▼ Become a member of the governor's health care advisory council.

▼ Become the medical commentator/adviser to a local television and radio station.

▼ Take a leadership role on a task force or committee in a state or national professional association.

▼ Volunteer medical services at a state, national, or international nonprofit organization.

▼ Become a medical adviser to a wilderness or luxury travel company.

▼ Accept locum tenens placement nationally or internationally, from prison settings to cruise ships.

▼ Volunteer to be the physician at major nonprofessional sports events.

▼ Volunteer in community public health projects (eg, depression screening, blood drives).

▼ Take an evening class at college or graduate school.

▼ Consult to a health care Web site as a freelance writer.

The possibilities for career diversification are endless. Once you decide to dedicate the requisite time and energy, the options are limited only by your creativity, resourcefulness, and spirit of adventure.

◪ Case Study

Dr X: Resourcefulness in the Diversification Process

It can be especially challenging when the new professional skills you wish to learn lie in nontraditional arenas. Yet those who are clear on what they are seeking, and intent on obtaining such skills, will find a way—even if it means leaving mainstream pathways.

Dr X was a primary care physician based at a community hospital affiliated with a major academic center in New York City. She became increasingly frustrated by the sense that she could not relieve the symptoms for an increasing number of her patients through traditional medical skills alone.

She became interested in acupuncture and wanted to learn how to develop the expertise necessary to incorporate it into her practice. Unable to find traditional CME courses that would provide this training, she made a number of contacts and eventually found her way to a practitioner in Chinatown. This very experienced practitioner eagerly agreed to take her on as an apprentice in acupuncture two half-days per week while Dr X continued to maintain her active clinical practice.

Chapter 6

Networking

This book simply would not be complete without a chapter on networking. Many physicians cringe at the very word because it elicits associations with all that is negative about the world of business. The term *networking* is used loosely, but I think of it as an "ongoing process of actively reaching out to meet new people."

Whatever its connotations, one thing is clear: The art of networking is essential for physicians to master as an integral element of strategic career management. (This is particularly true if one wants to pursue a nontraditional career path.)

The goals you should strive for while networking are:

▼ Cultivating new relationships

▼ Learning about the professional worlds of those you meet

▼ Identifying potential areas for formal or informal collaboration

Done well, networking can lead to new consulting and/or employment opportunities. However, this should not be your primary reason for doing it. Instead, networking should be approached as a wonderful way to learn about areas in health care (or other) industries that lie beyond your experience and awareness. In the process you'll meet people who can help you expand your contacts as your interests and activities evolve.

Networking is anything *but* one-sided. You, too, represent a potentially valuable resource to those you meet, so it is important that you be willing to reciprocate. If you develop a reputation as a "taker," rather than a "sharer," your ability to network will be drastically diminished. Whether it's a colleague, a medical student, or a medical device salesperson, spend whatever time you can building relationships with them.

Questions about Networking from Peers and Clients

Q: Why is networking so unappealing or intimidating to physicians?

A: Networking is not really a part of the medical culture in the same way it is a part of the business culture. In business, people tend to make more career transitions, and these transitions are often done through informal networking.

In medicine, individuals make fewer transitions over the course of their careers. Most of these occur after completing formal academic training with subsequent certification. For physicians, each career transition is more formal and structured. In business, career transitions tend to be more fluid, often facilitated by being in the right place at the right time and knowing the right people (another important function of skilled networking).

In addition, in the medical culture physicians generally learn not to speak up until [he or she] is considered expert on the subject. This communication model represents the antithesis of the networking process, which by definition requires initiating conversations with people you don't know about things you don't know much about.

Many physicians assume that a phone call that's not intended to accomplish a specific objective or answer a specific question will likely be viewed as a burdensome interruption. Perhaps because physicians receive so many uninvited solicitations from vendors, they don't want to be perceived in the same way. But what many physicians do not realize is that a *well-targeted* introduction to someone actually may be of value to the person being contacted because of the physician's expertise or perspectives. If your call is not well received or the person sounds annoyed, don't be offended. Simply chalk it up as something that goes with the territory of networking. You need to be able to deal with such rudeness and rejection and not take it personally. Above all, do *not* avoid networking if this happens or simply because you fear it *might* happen.

Q: Do I really have to network in order to make a career transition?

A: Yes. In fact, you should not wait until you are ready to make the transition to begin your networking. The real answer to this question is that you need to network *all the time* to actively manage your career in the current environment of medicine and industry. You should integrate networking into ongoing career activities at every opportunity.

Networking is not opportunistic, but it does create opportunities. Keep in mind that the contacts you make when you are happily employed often lead to new and exciting career developments. This is precisely because these conversations occur in relaxed, unpressured situations.

In advanced stages of your career, opportunities frequently come through networking rather than formal job postings or recruiters. It is not uncommon for a new job to be created specifically for you if you happen to speak with someone with hiring authority who thinks the chemistry is just right.

The bottom line is that the less traditional your career path, the more important it is that you become skilled at networking.

Networking

By William Lloyd, MD

William Lloyd, MD, an ophthalmologist from Texas, is one of MD IntelliNet's star networkers. His thoughts about networking are worthy of attention.

Just like the full scope of career management activities, the concept of networking is not confined to job-hunting. Networking can be effectively applied to locate needed office personnel, to obtain discount financing for new equipment, and to promote your practice throughout your community. It is a learned skill that improves with continued effort.

Doctor, why are you networking?

Did you say "network" or "need work"? Many professionals are confused with the fundamental basics of networking. The core activity of networking is the exchange of information. Don't enter into a networking opportunity with immediate expectations of landing a new career or closing a major business transaction.

Networking is a means to an end. Networking is not negotiating. It's very insulting to approach a corporate decision maker about any business proposition that is normally handled by other corporate or hospital staff. Double the penalties for attempting this during a social function.

Approach networking as you would a patient

This point simply cannot be overemphasized. Learn all you can before any networking encounter. (*"Hmm . . . am I performing an appendectomy or a cholecystectomy?"*) A small amount of preparation will yield powerful results.

First, your contact will be tremendously impressed with your effort, which will leverage handsomely at decision time. As for you, preparation ensures that you will not waste any portion of your valuable encounter exhibiting your ignorance.

Who does research when there are 40 patients to see in an afternoon?

Surprise! You may need only five minutes to gather the essential information. Here's a great example. Not long ago I was promoting some medical writing to a large health-related Internet Web site.

Once the teleconference with the CEO was scheduled, I started surfing. A quick Internet search provided me with a complete biographical sketch of this man, including some regional magazine articles I had not previously read.

When the time came for our informational interview, I was well prepared. Before long the CEO asked why his business should consider our services instead of its usual in-house writers.

Nodding, I agreed that my proposal represented a radical departure from tradition, not unlike the way the CEO had restructured XYZ Co to make it the industry leader. He paused for what seemed an eternity, then volunteered, "Ooh, pretty sharp!" That first impression was galvanized in his mind and we clicked.

The first opportunity is your best opportunity

The canaliculus is the tiny conduit that directs tears from the eye to the nose. The first attempt to repair a lacerated canaliculus is most often the best (perhaps only) chance to correct the problem.

Similarly, for networking efforts to cultivate professional business relationships, they also require a positive first effort. Simple gestures such as good grooming, a firm handshake, and good eye contact are powerful, persuasive signals. Don't neglect them.

Set expectations and meet them

What do you hope to achieve by networking? Be sure you and your prospect both know specifically why you are meeting. Don't be coy or evasive. If you are exploring an office relocation, don't get bogged down talking about golf.

Anticipate the unexpected

Patients have stopped breathing while being refracted for new glasses. Are you ready to step in and save the day? At your first meeting your networking partner may be preoccupied with big problems, and you may not feel cordially received. Any chances for progress are slim.

Convert a potential disaster into a winning solution by graciously offering to reschedule the session. This demonstrates concern on your part, as well as the ability to put others' feelings above your own needs.

What happens if you strike gold? Be ready for success as well as disappointment. You may discover that this new member of your networking circle has many of the answers you need for a specific project. This is a wonderful resource that deserves great consideration. Follow up meetings with a handwritten note and, if applicable, a summary of points discussed, along with pertinent contact information: names, phone/fax numbers, e-mail addresses, etc.

And what if nothing happens? Even if your meeting fails to produce the results you intended, don't discount its future value. More than once, contacts and leads planted during a long-forgotten, and not immediately productive, meeting have blossomed into rewarding opportunities.

Never be afraid to ask for assistance

You've spent your career as part of a team, so don't change things now. It's okay to admit to inexperience or knowledge gaps while networking. If you had all the answers, you wouldn't need to meet in the first place!

Suppose you are unsure regarding insurance matters or bureaucratic regulations. A generous networker will bring you up to speed promptly. Such a response is a sign of genuine interest and maturity on their part. I've rarely been burned by those who demonstrate such sincerity.

Any Physician Can Become a Successful Networker

Kindness is a great door-opener

Whenever I attend social functions, I always carry two freshly pressed handkerchiefs. One is for my personal use. But the second handkerchief is ready for any emergency: a wine spill by the hostess, a dropped hors d'oeuvre on the designer dress worn by the mayor's wife.

The simple gesture of offering the clean hankie creates a bridge that will long be remembered. On several occasions I have been treated to second invitations for the purpose of receiving the cleaned handkerchief.

Always assume your counterpart is more knowledgeable than you

Physicians are particularly vulnerable to the misconception that, because they hold the venerable Doctor of Medicine degree, they gain some immediate advantage over their networking associate. This logic is contrary to the basic principles of networking: sharing information, freely exchanging contacts, building mutual respect.

Many business professionals freely exploit this folly when it comes time to negotiate. This is probably one reason so many physicians own ranch land.

◤ Case Study

Dr Y: Networking Success Story

What is particularly interesting about this client (a pediatrician) is that, when I first began working with him, he felt quite awkward about both the process of networking and using the Internet. He then became increasingly comfortable with both of these through his career transition planning. Ultimately, he gained a sense of mastery over these media—not only as a means of gathering information, but also as a platform for a new job.

This client shares his reflections on his professional values and objectives. It was becoming painfully evident to him that he could not achieve professional satisfaction practicing medicine in the current industry.

March 1999

I went into medicine to help people have a healthy life and to contribute to the betterment of society; to be part of a profession that emphasized continued learning over the course of one's career to improve the level of care given.

I tried to follow the managed care provider model. It just wasn't what I could do. I practiced as if I were the father of a sick child. I knew what kind of care I wanted my child to have.

I met with the pediatrician and his significant other during a career consultation session, and we subsequently communicated closely by e-mail. By the time we met, Dr Y had already taken a leave of absence from his job so he could reflect and plan his next career move. Whatever his ultimate plan, he wanted to incorporate some public sector work into it.

Beyond that, though, he had no idea how to explore his options and find his way to specific opportunities in his local geographic area. We spent a portion of the session talking about how to use the Internet to search for ideas and resources, as he had minimal experience with it.

Later in March 1999

I have been looking into various possibilities here. Thinking that medical directors of the city and county health departments in Northern Virginia are in a good position to know about openings involving special needs and underserved pediatric populations, I've written to them. They have not all replied yet; however, this is not developing into a gold mine.

By networking, I have discovered the Community Foundation of Greater Washington. It has a library in the city that maintains directories of nonprofit organizations, foundations, and associations, which I have reviewed for those whose emphasis fits my interests. There are so many with national offices in the District.

My plan is to make telephone contact and visit people who will agree to see me. Additionally, I have found a couple of clinics here that provide free medical care to patients (including pediatrics) and residential facilities serving at-risk pediatric groups who need physicians to volunteer. I can work part-time while looking for salaried opportunities. As you see, I am gravitating to clinical positions.

May 1999

Greetings! I am happy to inform you that I have been hired to work with a company on the Internet. It is America's Doctor Online, which is one of the health channels of America Online.

They employ primary care physicians to conduct real-time chats with subscribers of AOL. Doctors and pharmacists work shifts to provide 24-hour coverage. Questions are answered in a general manner, without trying to make diagnoses. I am excited about this new opportunity.

Additionally, I will volunteer as a clinician at one of the free clinics in the area.

Dr Y found his way to this opportunity by answering an advertisement in the employment section of the *Washington Post* and attending an orientation session to learn more about it.

◣ Collateral Marketing Materials

As you network, you may want to develop collateral marketing materials to enhance the process. There is no standard procedure for this, so feel free to be creative. Some items you might want to consider include the following.

▼ A curriculum vitae revised from the traditional chronological format to more of a functional format or, as they call it in the business world, a resume. (*Note:* Rather than focus further on this topic here, refer to the other resources listed at the end of this chapter that amply address it.)

▼ Alternatively, or in addition to a resume, you might want to consider creating a biographical sketch. This type of document provides more of a story line, which can help "connect the dots" of one's nontraditional career path. You may want several versions of your resume or biographical sketch—each one emphasizing different aspects of your career to a specific target market.

▼ A new business card that introduces you as other than a full-time clinician. This card typically will have a brief byline that defines your new identity.

▼ A Web site that provides key highlights, such as your contact information, resume, or biographical sketch, and copies of any articles you have written (published or not).

Your ability to refine your collateral marketing materials for maximum impact will improve tremendously as your networking and market research proceed. The knowledge you gain through these activities will help you use these marketing materials to position yourself for success.

References

American Medical Association. *Leaving the Bedside: The Search for a Nonclinical Career.* Chicago, Ill: American Medical Association; 1993.

Asher D. *Asher's Bible of Executive Resumes and How to Write Them.* Berkeley, Calif: Ten Speed Press; 1996.

Boe A, Youngs BB. *Is Your "Net" Working?: A Complete Guide to Building Contacts and Career Visibility.* New York, NY: John Wiley & Sons Inc; 1989.

Fish D. *People Power: 12 Power Principles to Enrich Your Business, Career & Personal Networks.* Austin, Tex: Bard Press; 1995.

Gladwell M. Six Degrees of Lois Weisberg. *New Yorker.* January 11, 1999:53-63.

Heenehan M. Networking. *Princeton Rev.* 1997(Job Notes Series).

Krannich RL, Krannich C, Banis WJ. *High Impact Resumes and Letters : How to Communicate Your Qualifications to Employers.* 7th ed. Manassas Park, Va: Impact Publications; 1998.

Pack T. *10 Minute Guide to Business Research on the Net.* Indianapolis, Ind: Que Education and Training; 1997.

Rockport Publishers, compiler. *The Best of Business Card Design 3.* Gloucester, Mass: Rockport Publishers; 1998.

Shaw PD, Landmann PC. *Web Site Planning and Design Workbook.* Assets Protection; 1997.

Chapter 7

Navigating Vertical Market Sectors

In Chapter 5 we discussed the importance of creating a personalized plan for diversifying your career or making a major transition. One of the key elements of that plan relates to the process by which you define your direction. This chapter will provide an overview of some of the key health care market sectors that lie outside of patient care and offer suggestions about how to go about exploring them.

In strategic career planning, the process is "marketplace driven." This simply means your plan should be shaped by *knowledge* of current industry trends—whether it's administration, pharmaceuticals, equipment, or devices. But therein lies the challenge. The very words, *marketplace driven*, represent a foreign concept to most physicians.

Most career and outplacement counselors have their client focus on his or her values, priorities, motivations, and strengths. Further vocational testing can pinpoint known types of traditional jobs and discern the potential for a fit between the individual and such jobs. Armed with that insight, the individual and his or her counselor then can develop action plans for approaching companies that might have the kinds of jobs that interest the physician.

Certainly these insights about oneself and the traditional job market are important for physicians to understand. However, these tools are not enough to help one clearly define one's target companies and jobs in the current health care market. The challenge these days is that the health care industry is changing at lightning speed. Physicians are playing many new roles that didn't even exist as recently as 5 or 10 years ago. Many of the best diversification positions for physicians are not represented in standard vocational interest tests because they are such new career categories. Some of these roles are being defined—and redefined—day by day in the current industry.

In addition, emerging areas of the nonclinical marketplace may offer new opportunities that can be difficult to find through traditional job-hunting channels. Indeed, it is very nearly a full-time job today just to stay on top of those health care market trends that might have important implications for physician careers. Thus, the ideal approach for finding a position outside your current arena is to combine traditional career counseling tools (develop insight into what makes you tick and where your strengths lie) with information gleaned from your market research efforts.

You may well be saying, "I'm a physician, not a pollster! How do I do market research?" It's somewhat challenging because there is no central repository of market data where you can obtain a coordinated, organized presentation of the major market sectors in health care. There is no list of information about roles and specific opportunities for physicians. One of the things MD IntelliNet has done is begin to build such a database, so our clients can be apprised of the latest market-based research and information about the burgeoning careers that are opening almost daily to the well-prepared physician.

Some Major Market Sectors in Health Care and Where Physicians May Fit

Pharmaceuticals

Biotechnology

Medical Devices

▼ Clinical research

▼ Outcomes research

▼ Marketing and sales

▼ Medical affairs

▼ Regulatory affairs

▼ Program officer/director of foundation

Information Technology

▼ Content research and development

▼ Product development

▼ Product marketing

▼ Product management

▼ Sales

▼ Systems implementation

▼ Information systems management

Business/Management

▼ Management consulting

▼ Medical management

▼ Operations management

▼ Executive management

▼ Entrepreneurship

▼ Business development

Insurance (eg, life, health, disability, malpractice)

▼ Underwriting

▼ Claims management

▼ Utilization review

▼ Risk appraisal and management

▼ Actuarials

▼ Independent medical evaluations

▼ Benefits consulting

Finance

▼ Venture capital

▼ Investment banking

▼ Investment analysis consulting

▼ Financial planning and management

Law

▼ Independent medical evaluation/expert witness

▼ Technology transfer

▼ Forensics

▼ Mediation/Arbitration

▼ Regulatory compliance

Policy

▼ Professional and trade associations

▼ Think tanks

▼ Interest groups

▼ Congress and congressional agencies

▼ Federal agencies

Public Health

▼ Public health service

▼ Quantitative and qualitative research

▼ Epidemiology

▼ Preventive medicine

▼ International health

Marketing and Communications

▼ Corporate communications

▼ Market research

▼ Multimedia publishing

▼ Advertising

▼ Sales

▼ Educational programs (for professionals and patients)

▼ Information/Knowledge management

▼ Broadcast journalism (television, cable, and radio)

A physician can do many things on his or her own to learn more about a targeted market sector:

▼ Identify professional associations related to your area of interest. Find such associations through professional journals or Internet key word searches. Most associations these days have extensive Web sites (though the most helpful information is often reserved for members). Or simply ask around; search the phone book and local business publications.

▼ Join appropriate associations to get on the right mailing lists and subscription base for any information about helpful resources and opportunities.

▼ Consider related trade associations as a means of learning about broader business and policy issues. Attend their annual conferences and read their publications.

▼ Establish a community of peers with shared interests. One way to do this is to scan membership directories from relevant associations for potential contact information.

▼ If you can find a physician working in a company that might be desirable to you, contact him or her directly. Establishing such peer-to-peer contacts is far better than making cold calls to human resource personnel, who usually won't give you the time of day.

▼ Don't forget about trade publications that can broaden your perspective on medical issues and health care market trends (eg, *The Wall Street Journal, Healthcare Business, Forbes*, and *Inc.* magazine, to name a few).

▼ Join local social and service clubs to network with nonphysicians who share your evolving interests. For example, I live in Boston and have found that the MIT Enterprise Forum (http://www.mitforum-cambridge.org) is a great way to meet people interested in technology and entrepreneurship).

▼ Visit amazon.com's Web site (http://www.amazon.com) and search for books on topics related to the market sector. (More on this at the end of this chapter.)

▼ Search the Internet for companies in the market sector you're interested in and check their site for job postings to learn more about qualifications sought and salary ranges. Add the most interesting sites to your "bookmarks" or "favorites" list to easily monitor the latest postings. When you visit these sites, look for any e-mail contacts who are available to provide more information.

▼ Seek out educational courses that provide the skill sets you need to develop. Such courses may be available through academic institutions, professional associations, or training organizations. One such training organization— PERI, or the Pharmaceutical Education and Research Institute (www.peri.org)—provides seminars that target specific commercial skills needed within the pharmaceutical industry, as opposed to academic courses. Whether such courses offer CME credit is irrelevant. What you want is information. Some training organizations also offer a degree track that would increase your marketability.

▼ Reentering the classroom provides the opportunity to make new contacts in your target market sector. Use this strategy to learn as much as possible about where faculty and the other students work. Set up informational interviews. (Don't forget the thank you note!) Distribute those new business cards, and let your new contacts know they also can call on you for assistance.

▼ Join a relevant committee in your hospital or managed care organization (eg, technology assessment or utilization review/quality improvement). This is a great way to meet new colleagues and even vendors. Committee membership is also an excellent way to learn more about the business perspectives of clinical issues.

The bottom line is this: You must be *active, strategic,* and *aggressive* when it comes to gathering information about a target market sector that will enhance your career.

◢ Case Study

Dr S: Against the Odds

When I asked one of my clients if it was all right to use an excerpt from one of his e-mail messages to me, he wrote back to say he wanted to expand on this message. To me the point of his story is how resourceful some physicians can be, despite enormous odds. Through aggressive networking they *can* leverage professional skills, experiences, and contacts to create new opportunities.

To protect his privacy, Dr S is intentionally vague about the companies he's talked to and the roles he plays. However, he stresses to his colleagues reading this that it *is* possible to reshape a career midstream.

I am an internist in a busy subspecialty practice and have developed paraplegia (walking disability) after 30 years of practice. The physical demands of full-time private practice made it impossible for me to continue. I successfully managed the transformation from physician to business consultant and now write and edit articles about my subspecialty for various companies and consulting agencies.

I also work as a consultant for a company that reviews hospital programs in my field and have been able to market my medical training, knowledge, and experience successfully as a consultant for physician groups and hospitals.

I became administrator of a program in my specialty (vice president of medical affairs) and spent a year in business school to upgrade the informal business experience I gained in practice. I opened a small office to see only second-opinion referrals in my specialty, and am sought after because I'm not in competition with practicing physicians.

Various other companies and businesses, governmental agencies (eg, the FDA), and attorneys have sought my services as a consultant, and I have worked with insurance companies doing utilization review and quality assurance consultations.

I continue to write articles for the medical literature and have written a best-selling book for the public about my subspecialty. Most recently I have begun work as a business consultant and planner for a hospital system. This allows me to use my medical and business expertise in a novel and useful way.

Web Site Addresses Referenced in This Book

The Internet is a tremendously powerful facilitator of the market research and networking activities integral to strategic management of your medical career. As your interests become more focused, you can do key word searches that allow you to find relevant resources without having to first know their exact name and location.

The Internet is so powerful, in fact, that those who do not use it on a regular basis in their career management are at a distinct disadvantage. Consequently, we have tried to provide Web site addresses—or URLs—for all of the major organizational resources mentioned in this book.

If you would like to become more facile in your use of the Internet, contact the American Medical Association to obtain a list of CME programs they offer for this purpose.

Note: Standard URL formatting is implied for all of the addresses listed below unless otherwise indicated. In other words, www.amazon.com implies that the full address would be http://www.amazon.com.

Professional and Trade Associations

Academy of Occupational and Organizational Psychiatry
www.mcn.com.aoop.htm

American Academy of Insurance Medicine
www.aaimedicine.org

American Academy of Pharmaceutical Physicians
www.aapp.org

American College of Healthcare Executives
www.ache.org

American College of Legal Medicine
www.aclm.org

American College of Physician Executives
www.acpe.org

American Medical Association
www.ama-assn.org

American Medical Directors Association
www.amda.org

American Medical Informatics Association
www.amia.org

American Public Health Association
www.apha.org

American Society of Law, Medicine, and Ethics
www.aslme.org

American Telemedicine Association
www.atmeda.org

Association for the Advancement of Medical Instrumentation
www.aami.org

Association of Health Services Research
www.ahsr.org

Association of Management Consulting Firms
www.amcf.org

Association of Medical Directors of Information Systems
www.amdis.org

Drug Information Association
www.diahome.org

Healthcare Information Management Society
www.himss.org

Healthcare Marketing and Communication Council
www.hmc-council.org

Health Industry Manufacturers Association
www.himanet.com

Health Insurance Association of America
www.hiaa.org

Institute of Management Consultants
www.imcusa.org

Medical Marketing Association
www.mmanet.org

National Association of Healthcare Consultants
www.healthcon.org

National Association of Pharmaceutical Manufacturers
http://www.napmnet.org

National Health Lawyers Association
www.nhla.org

Pharmaceutical Research and Manufacturers of America
www.phrma.org

Other

Amazon.com
www.amazon.com
On-line bookstore that can be very useful in your research of different health care market sectors.

CenterWatch
www.centerwatch.com
Publishing company that focuses on the clinical trials industry.

Health Data Management Resource Guide
http://hdm.fgray.com/html/buyers/main.htm
Annual catalog of major companies that operate in health care information technology. This resource can help you understand the full range of products that exist within this sector, as well as provide you with contact information for specific companies.

MIT Enterprise Forum
www.mitforum-cambridge.org
Club that focuses on technology entrepreneurship.

MD IntelliNet (formerly MD CareerNet)
www.mdintellinet.com
Web site for the company founded and headed by this book's author. It provides career resource information and services to physicians.

Medical Device Link
www.devicelink.com
Major marketing and information channel for the medical device industry.

Pharmaceutical Education and Research Institute
www.peri.org
Training company that specializes in practical courses for those who work in the pharmaceutical industry.

◆ Exploring the Commercial Market

At a certain point in your exploration of target markets, it becomes important to learn more about specific companies in that sector. Here's how you go about doing this.

Identify Major Companies in Your Target Market Sector

The major companies usually have a vendor's booth or are a corporate sponsor at annual conferences of those professional or trade organizations you are most interested in. Take advantage of these conferences to make contacts at these companies.

Again, use those all-important Internet key word searches. Identify key online marketing channels for industry sectors. Examples include:

Medical Device Link (www.devicelink.org)

Health Data Management Resource Guide
(http://hdm.fgray.com/html/buyers/main.htm)

From these centralized marketing channel sites, you can hyperlink directly to the Web sites of your companies of interest to learn more about them. Those of greatest interest can be further studied by sending an e-mail to request a corporate information packet.

Study job postings on each Web site. In addition to finding some that may interest you, you'll learn what roles exist in that market sector, position titles and salary ranges, qualifications sought for each position, etc.

Contacting Companies

If you find a job posting on a company's Web site that looks like a good fit, you should follow the instructions provided for interested candidates. In most cases, though, human resource personnel are flooded with resumes. So it may be to your advantage to find more creative ways to make contact with the company. For example, contact any individuals you know personally or professionally who now work, or have worked, for the company. See if they can give you the name and phone number, or e-mail address, of someone there who might be in a position to help you. When possible, try to make contact with a physician working in the company. Although he or she may not have hiring authority, because you are peers he or she might give you inside information about how the company is organized and what persons to contact.

Keep in mind that many companies in your target sector receive a substantial number of unsolicited phone calls from physicians seeking a nonclinical employment opportunity. So it's important to do your homework before you make any cold calls. Be prepared to provide a succinct statement about why you are calling, ideally one that will catch their interest in 30 to 60 seconds.

Suggestions for Developing an Effective Telephone Contact

Again, do your homework on the company. Make it clear you are not calling *every* company in that market sector. Rather, emphasize that you have studied the market and there is a *specific* reason you are calling them. Then tell them that reason.

Suggest that you have specific ideas that may help them enter a new market or find a new application for their product. Particularly if the company is a start-up or is preparing to launch a new product, express interest in seeing their services or product firsthand.

Then try to arrange a time to meet with representatives of the company at their office. With this approach you let them know you have something of value for them, rather than simply calling to ask for a job or consulting opportunity.

It is important not to mislead, however. If you are under immediate pressure to find a job and use this oblique approach, the individual you contact may resent that you did not go through proper channels.

Again, this "informational" approach is best used when you have time for a more leisurely networking process. Occasionally this approach will lead to a consulting opportunity, but it is best not to go into it with that expectation. If you secure a visit to the company, your primary goals are to learn as much about them as possible and to build new relationships.

Visiting the Company

Leave them with your business card and resume, as well as any articles or other materials you've written that deal directly with their subject area. Follow up with a brief thank you note.

Stay in touch with your contact. For example, if you come across an article relevant to what the two of you discussed, forward it with a brief update of your situation. Go up to say hello if you see him or her at a conference or the like.

While seemingly simplistic, these tips are among the most often cited things business executives tell me physicians do wrong when attempting to build relationships with their organizations.

The art of networking, which is often a foreign skill for physicians, is subtlety at its finest. Think of it as part Emily Post, part Golden Rule, part doing what your mother taught you about good manners, and part common sense. Even if you believe you shouldn't have to participate in these niceties, remember that physicians who *do* move on in their careers are probably practicing these business/social graces. That alone should be impetus to do likewise.

◤ A Virtual Trip Through the Vertical Market Sectors of Health Care

As you explore vertical market sectors within the health care industry, one exercise that can be useful as well as fun is to browse through the amazon.com Web site. By doing key word searches in areas of evolving interest to you, you can broaden your understanding of specific niches within these sectors. Even if you do not purchase any of the books, simply learning about the topics represented can help you lay out your personal map of the health care marketplace. What follows are some sample books identified by doing such market-specific key word searches on the amazon.com Web site.

Healthcare Business and Management

Physician Equity Groups and Other Emerging Equity: Competitive Organizational Choices for Physicians (HFMA–Healthcare Financial Management Series)
Fred, PhD McCall-Perez / Hardcover / Published 1997

IPA, PHO MSO Development Strategies: Building Successful Provider Alliances
Maria K. Todd / Hardcover / Published 1997

Med Inc: How Consolidation Is Shaping Tomorrow's Healthcare System. (Jossey-Bass Health Series)
Sandy Lutz et al / Hardcover / Published 1998

Capitation in California: A Study of Physician Organizations Managing Risk
Maurice J. Penner / Paperback / Published 1997

Management for Hospital Doctors
Maurice Burrows et al / Hardcover / Published 1994

Medical Group Management in Turbulent Times: How Physician Leadership Can Optimize Health Plan, Hospital, and Medical Group Performance
Paul A. Sommers / Hardcover / Published 1998

Physician Driven Health Plans
William J. Demarco, Kenneth M. Hekman / Hardcover / Published 1998

Physician Practice Management Redefined
John F. McCally, Michel A. Lafond / Hardcover / Published 1998

Rethinking Health Care: Innovation and Change in America
Max Heirich / Hardcover / Published 1998

The Physician Strategist: Setting a Strategic Direction for Your Practice
Linda E. Swayne et al / Hardcover / Published 1996

A Guide to Consulting Services for Emerging Healthcare Organizations
Robert James Cimasi / Hardcover / Published 1999

1999 Career Guide: Management Consulting (Harvard Business School Career Guides)
Neil Nunn, ed, et al / Paperback / Published 1998

The 1999 WetFeet Insider Guide: So, You Want to Be a Management Consultant
Wet Feet Press, ed / Spiral-bound / Published 1999

The Business of Consulting: The Basics and Beyond
Elaine Biech / Hardcover / Published 1998

Health Care Finance

*Financial Analysis and Decision
Making for Healthcare Organizations:
A Guide for the Healthcare Professional*
Louis C. Gapenski / Hardcover /
Published 1997

*The 1998 WetFeet Insider Guide to Jobs
in Venture Capital*
Wet Feet Press / Spiral Bound /
Published 1998

*The 1999 WetFeet Insider Guide: So,
You Want to Be an Investment Banker*
Gary Alpert / Wet Feet Press / Spiral
Bound / Published 1999

*The Funding of Young Investigators in
the Biological and Biomedical Sciences*
Shirley M. Tilghman, Torsten N.
Wiesel / Paperback / Published 1994

*Funding Health Sciences Research: A
Strategy to Restore Balance*
Floyd E. Bloom, Mark A. Randolph,
ed / Hardcover / Published 1991

*Successful Grant Writing: Strategies for
Health and Human Service*
Laura N. Gitlin, Kevin J. Lyons /
Paperback / Published 1996

*Capitation : New Opportunities in
Healthcare Delivery*
David I. Samuels / Hardcover /
Published 1996

*Health Care Innovation and Venture
Trends*
Courtney Price / Hardcover /
Published 1992

*Physician's Financial Sourcebook:
Investment, Risk Management &
Retirement Tools for a Balanced Life*
Paul H. Sutherland / Paperback /
Published 1998

Health Care Law and Policy

*Effective Medical Testifying: A
Handbook for Physicians*
William T. Tsushima, PhD, Kenneth
K. Nakano, MD / Paperback /
Published 1998

*Legal Aspects of Health Information
Management*
(Health Information Management
Series)
Dana C. McWay / Hardcover /
Published 1996

*Legal Check-Up for Medical Practice:
Essential Guide for the Health Care Team*
Salvatore Francis Fiscina et al /
Paperback / Published 1997

*Criminalistics: An Introduction to
Forensic Science*
Richard Saferstein / Hardcover /
Published 1997

*Complementary & Alternative
Medicine: Legal Boundaries and
Regulatory Perspectives*
Michael H. Cohen / Hardcover /
Published 1999

*Telemedicine in Hospitals: Issues in
Implementation*
(Health Care Policy in the United
States)
Sherry Emery / Hardcover /
Published 1998

Information Technology

*Introduction to Clinical Informatics
(Computers in Health Care)*
Patrice Degoulet, Benjamin Phister,
translator, Marius Fieschi
contributor / Hardcover /
Published 1996

*Clinical Decision Support Systems:
Theory and Practice (Health
Informatics)*
Eta S. Berner, M. J. Ball, eds /
Hardcover / Published 1998

*The Computer-Based Patient Record:
An Essential Technology for
Health Care*
(Institute of Medicine) Elaine B.
Steen, Richard S. Dick, eds /
Hardcover / Published 1998

*Dealing With Medical Knowledge :
Computers in Clinical Decision Making*
(The Language of Science)
Tibor Deutsch, Ewart Carson, Endre
Ludwig / Harcover / Published 1995

*Ethics, Computing, and Medicine:
Informatics and the Transformation of
Health Care*
Kenneth W. Goodman, ed /
Hardcover / 1998

*How to Find Health Information on
the Internet*
Bruce Maxwell / Paperback /
Published 1998

*Planning and Implementing Your
Health Care Internet Strategy*
Edward Fotsch, Ron Wolf /
Paperback / Published 1996

*Home Healthcare: Wired and Ready for
Telemedicine*
Audrey Kinsella / Paperback /
Published 1997

*Telemedicine: Practicing in the
Information Age*
Steven F. Viegas, MD, Kim Dunn, MD,
PhD, eds / Paperback / Published 1998

Medical Devices

*Sources of Medical Technology:
Universities and Industry*
(Medical Innovation at the
Crossroads, Vol. 5)
Nathan Rosenberg, et al, eds /
Paperback / Published 1994

*Clinical Evaluation of Medical Devices:
Principles and Case Studies*
Karen Becker Witkin, ed / Hardcover /
Published 1997

*Creating Technology Strategies:
How to Build Competitive
Biomedical R&D*
Alice M. Sapienza / Paperback /
Published 1997

*Medical Device Accidents: With
Illustrative Cases*
Leslie A. Geddes / Hardcover /
Published 1998

*Biomedical and Clinical
Instrumentation: Fast Tracking from
Concept Through Production in a
Regulated Environment*
Robert Meltzer / Hardcover /
Published 1994

*Small Business Innovation Research
Grants—1998 (Including Fast-Track
SBIRs)*
Michael G. Pappas, Alexandra F.
Pappas / Ring-bound / Published 1998

Pharmaceuticals and Biotechnology

Careers in Clinical Research: Obstacles and Opportunities
William N. Kelley, Mark A. Randolph, eds / Hardcover / Published 1994

Discovering New Medicines: Careers in Pharmaceutical Research and Development
Peter D. Stonier, ed / Paperback / Published 1995

The Physician's Guide to Clinical Research Opportunities: How to Create a Rewarding Business and Professional Relationship Between Your Medical Practice . . .
Matthew D.Heller, MD, James A. Boyle, MD / Paperback / Published 1996

References

Ginsberg D, Whitaker R. *The Investigator's Guide to Clinical Research.* Boston, Mass: CenterWatch; 1997.

Robbins-Roth C. *Alternative Careers in Science: Leaving the Ivory Tower.* San Diego, Calif: Academic Press; 1993.

Chapter 8

Industry's Perspective

I wish to thank the following individuals and their organizations for their willingness to participate in the development of this book. Without their assistance, this book would be a lesser project.

John Abele
Founder and Chairman
Boston Scientific Corporation
Watertown, MA

David Boyko, MD
Vice President, US Medical Affairs
Glaxo Wellcome
Research Triangle Park, NC

Rebecca Campen, MD, JD
Chief of Staff,
Department of Dermatology
Massachusetts General Hospital
Boston, MA

Ed Erickson, PhD
Division Vice President,
Medical-Surgical Division
3M Corporation
St Paul, MN

Robert Gussin, PhD
Corporate Vice President,
Science and Technology
Chief Scientific Officer
Johnson & Johnson
New Brunswick, NJ

Tony Imondi, PhD
Vice President of Oncology Franchise
Battelle
Columbus, OH

Pat Jamieson, MD
Product Manager,
Knowledge-Based Systems
Cerner Corporation
Kansas City, MO

Ron Keeney, MD
Director of Clinical Research
Wake Medical Clinical
Research Institute
University of North Carolina
School of Medicine
Raleigh, NC

Samuel Langstaff, MD, MBA
Principal
Carolina Financial Securities, LLC
Westminster, CO

Steve McGeady
Vice President, New Business Group
Director, Internet Health Initiative
Intel Corporation
Hillsboro, OR

Richard Moscicki, MD
Chief Medical Officer
Senior Vice President for Clinical
Regulatory Medical Affairs
Genzyme Inc
Cambridge, MA

Tom Reichert, MD, PhD
Vice President of
Quantitative Planning
Beckton Dickinson and Company
Franklin Lakes, NJ

Marshall Stanton, MD
Vice President of Medical Affairs,
Cardiac Rhythm Management Division
Medtronic
Minneapolis, MN

Steve Tuel, MD, MBA
Vice President, Business Development
Luna Innovations, Inc
Blacksburg, VA

◭ Introduction

As physicians, we control or influence $800 billion in annual health care expenditures. Yet to the business world, we represent one of the least well-understood market segments. Attempts by those on the business side of health care to influence, manage, or collaborate with physicians are fraught with tremendous frustration.

One need not spend more than a few minutes with executives from the pharmaceutical, medical device, or other such organizations that sell products and services to physicians before the "war stories" are trotted out with gusto. It's clear that, although most of these executives speak favorably and with fondness about their personal physicians, as a professional group we have a very serious public relations problem, especially when it comes to being hired in the business world.

Health care companies both within and outside of the clinical services sector have a variety of relationships with physicians. Physicians may be:

customers,

end-users of products,

sources of market research data,

expert consultants and advisory board members,

employees,

business development partners, or

providers of care to employees and their families.

Whatever the relationship, its context has altered dramatically in the past 10 to 15 years. Specifically, the forces of managed care have converged to create a chaotic, rapidly changing environment where long-standing tensions between physicians and industry are exacerbated. Yet at the same time, new opportunities emerge almost daily for those physicians and industry leaders willing to consider them.

🖎 Physicians as Employees

When asked why they chose to become a doctor, most physicians cite as key reasons their desire to help others and to have autonomy, respect, and security (both job and financial). Indeed, when they committed to their medical training, there was an implicit psychological contract. In exchange for approximately 10 years of dedicated time, energy, and resources, they would in turn receive the rewards they sought. In recent years, this psychological contract has been broken, leaving many physicians bitter and angry.

Most people outside medicine, especially those on the business end of health care, state emphatically that physicians themselves brought about this turn of events. They then proceed to offer countless illustrations of how this happened. Little is served by playing such "blame games." Regardless of who's responsible for the current state in medicine, the result is that more than half of a highly trained pool of professionals, accustomed to autonomy, have found themselves in the very unnatural role of employee. In most cases, this is at direct odds with their original career objectives.

When physicians become employees, certain behavioral and attitudinal traits tend to emerge that make them a challenge for managers. "Trying to manage physicians is like trying to herd cats," is how one physician executive put it. "They are arrogant, entitled, demanding and independent," said another. "Not team players," is the complaint of yet another business leader in the medical community. "They think they should get the same pay as the CEO, even though they've never worked in this industry sector before!" adds one hiring authority.

These frequent and consistent comments from managers in all health care market sectors, including physicians who have become managers, have led me to coin the term *cultural impairment syndrome* to encompass the array of unhelpful working styles, traits, and attitudes of physicians.

That said, some physicians thrive as employees, particularly in organizations where there are opportunities for their promotion into management positions. Today more than ever, physicians can move up the ladder into such roles.

🖎 Physicians in Business

Traditionally, fewer than 5% of all US physicians choose a career path that does not involve direct patient care. This is distinctly different from Europe, where 40% of medical school graduates choose a nonclinical path. This is likely related to differing educational systems. Physicians in Europe enter their medical training at an earlier age, when they may be less clear on their career goals. According to one industry executive, his company's success at recruiting physicians who make the transition from clinician to industrial employee has been much better with European physicians.

Yet typically a transition from clinical medicine to the business world carries a tremendous amount of soul searching for physicians. Those who grapple with this decision encounter a range of reactions from friends, colleagues, and career counselors. The sum and substance of their "advice" is that the physician should come to his or her senses and remain in clinical medicine for the following reasons:

▼ They should not abandon their colleagues and patients.

▼ Their move will represent a waste of national resources.[1]

▼ They've now reached the "top of the mountain."

▼ Their families sacrificed so much to make their medical training possible.

▼ They would be "selling out" to commercialism.

▼ Those who leave medicine tend to be itching to retire or unable to cope with clinical pressures. (Indeed, they may be impaired or have licensure restrictions.)

These notions are clearly beginning to change. It is increasingly acceptable, even highly desirable, for a physician to make the transition to industry.

"A move to pharmaceuticals no longer has the blemish it had ten to fifteen years ago. In fact, it is quite desirable now," says one physician in industry. "Most of my clinical colleagues were very supportive of my decision. Some were even envious.

"It used to be that the physicians who came into industry did so to get out of clinical medicine. They were of highly variable quality, professionally speaking. Starting in the late 70's we saw a change . . . an influx of very young, smart, dynamic physicians. They came because of the opportunities available to them here. There has been a growing awareness that research and development (R&D) can be just as good in industry as it is in academia.

"Doctors are beginning to recognize that R&D in industry may be more exciting—more cutting edge—than it is in academia. And that the intellectual challenges may be greater. I think this may be particularly true in biotech, where the companies may be smaller. Physicians may leave academia [for these companies] to play a range of very active roles and have access to greater resources."

Even more recently, those in industry are seeing an increased number of physicians with master's degrees in business administration (MBAs), whose interests extend beyond clinical trials to business development. "Some of these folks are

---

[1] Oransky I. An apology for those who leave medicine. *JAMA.* 1999;281:1230.

terrific. They are aggressive, know what the needs are and exactly where to look for things."

One pharmaceutical industry executive comments, "It used to be very uncommon for physicians to move from R&D into the commercial side of the business. This is changing as companies gain an appreciation that mastery of the 'technology' really is an important core competency for senior managers."

Many of those interviewed for this book see increased opportunities for physicians to play a broader range of roles in industry—particularly those who also have an MBA.

In the past a move from clinical medicine into industry tended to be more of a mid-career afterthought. Today some observers speculate that a future trend for the ambitious young person will be to get an MD degree as a "supplemental degree"—in other words, as a stepping-stone to an ultimate career goal in industry.

Although many physicians hope to find corporate employers who will fund their MBA training, such opportunities remain unusual, at least for now. And, although physicians who get MBAs do have increasing opportunities in industry, many physicians *and* nonphysicians acknowledge that a glass ceiling remains for MDs. This glass ceiling significantly limits access to roles for physicians in business and operations, even for those who obtain MBAs and other management degrees. The glass ceiling results from the long-held perception of those working in business roles within health care that "Once a physician, always a physician."

When I asked several industry executives for their reactions to this statement, here's what they said:

▼ "[It] may sound like an unfair stereotype; but even when they have an MBA, scratch the surface and you'll find the physician." (This from a physician executive!)

▼ One executive began by speaking enthusiastically about the broader range of opportunities for MDs with MBAs. He then chuckled and said, "Well you might be right. My wife is a physician and, even after getting her MBA, she remains a medical director." Still, this executive thinks there are more roles in industry for physicians with MBAs. He is actively involved at his company as a mentor to business-oriented physicians.

▼ "I never really thought about it before. But now that you mention it, the physicians here with MBAs are all in medical affairs."

When pushed on this point, industry executives once again referred to symptoms of the "cultural impairment syndrome." It is not difficult to gather from such remarks that those in industry perceive the negative traits ascribed to physicians as much like incurable genetic flaws, which are both fixed and fatal. This is important for physicians to recognize if they seek to move their careers in any nontraditional direction.

The result of such narrow-minded thinking on the part of industry is unfair, rigid pigeonholing of physicians. On the other hand, stereotypes generally evolve from at least some elements of truth. And, unfortunately, this is yet another affirmation of the business golden rule: He who has the gold rules.

◢ Medical Experience—Bonus or Baggage?

In addition to the cultural impairment syndrome that works against physicians, there is a lack of appreciation for how a physician's roles in medicine can transfer to management outside of medicine. One physician with an MBA spoke with me about his recent experience applying for a position within a venture capital firm. "I spoke with one partner [in the firm] who is an MD. He said he couldn't get his partners to understand how my experience building clinical and educational programs had anything to do with entrepreneurship." Even though in these programs he did in-depth market research, recruited and trained new staff, developed a new incentive structure for employees, worked closely with architects on the design of a new hospital, and developed the operational details of many new services, they still didn't see the relevance.

"All of this would have been considered 'business' experience if my title were Director of Business Development. But because it was Medical Director, no one could see how what I did was related to business."

Not only are physician management experiences not viewed by industry as transferable, the medical degree itself is often directly or indirectly held against physicians who want to make a career transition. One physician reports, "I got my MD, but didn't go into clinical practice. I had a tough time getting a job until I just dropped the MD from my resume. Suddenly I was 'very qualified' to do computer programming, whereas before no one would interview me for similar jobs."

◢ Medical vs Business Lexicon

One other trait of the cultural impairment syndrome that serves as a serious barrier to alternative career transitions for physicians is their tendency to use medical jargon in conversation. Although this may be appropriate when speaking with medical colleagues, it probably only intimidates and confuses those outside of the profession. One physician with an MBA who recently applied for a job in an investment banking firm said, "I knew I had no chance with them when one of the partners asked me if I knew a particular venture capitalist who is an MD. He then said, 'I can't understand half of what he says.'"

Furthermore, some business executives say that by getting an MBA, physicians are not only unsuccessful at gaining acceptance by their business colleagues, but they *also* lose their membership in the physician's "club." "I am a now a Dr to my business colleagues and a Mr to my physician colleagues," says one frustrated physician.

◆ Increasing Number of Roles, but Selectivity Is Increasing, Too

Physicians not interested in R&D or getting an MBA should be heartened to learn that there are an increasing number of roles for them in peer-to-peer product marketing and sales, particularly in the information technology (IT) sector. Many physicians seeking a transition into industry may not be interested in such roles, however, because they tend not to be comfortable in marketing and sales.

In addition, sales positions typically provide reduced salaries for physicians because some of the compensation package is performance based. Also, some physicians working in these roles may become frustrated that their clinical knowledge is not really valued, and they may become intellectually bored and frustrated.

That said, when the fit is right, placing a physician in sales can be a highly successful move, both for the physician and the company. More physicians than ever before are interested in such roles, particularly those who have successfully integrated specific IT products into their practice—and recognize the value of these tools. "I was reluctant to spend the time learning to use our new electronic medical record, and so were most of my colleagues. But once I decided to go for it, and after I got through the initial frustration, I saw how it revolutionized our ability to care for our patients. Now I want to help other docs get on board!" says one physician who called MD IntelliNet when looking for an opportunity to join an IT company in a marketing and sales role.

One industry physician comments that when he made the transition from academia into the computer industry in 1993, he was 1 of 4 physicians in the company. He remains with the same company today but is now 1 of 20 physician employees. Although companies in the IT sector increasingly recognize the potential value of physician employees, they are becoming increasingly selective in their hiring practices. "It is difficult now to be hired into the industry without an additional degree, like in medical informatics or public health," reports this same physician.

Another phenomenon is that—despite the number of MDs in industry increasing on the macro level—in most companies the number of openings for physicians is still quite small. Taking the organizations represented by the executives I interviewed as a starting point, the numbers look like this:

▼ Device company—12 physicians out of 17,000 total employees

▼ Biotech firm—15 physicians out of 3,500 total employees

One executive comments that his company still doesn't understand the importance of the clinician's perspective in the product development process.

Selectivity on the part of pharmaceutical companies also is increasing, according to executive recruiters. There is an increasing trend toward requiring physician candidates to have some prior industry experience, though not too much. "The ideal candidate will have had two to three years of experience in the pharmaceutical industry. That way the companies don't have to start from scratch in training them, but they also don't have to pay them that much either!" Another executive notes, "In the past we used to insist that physicians who wanted to become employees here had not worked with any of our competitors. Now we recognize that those who have worked with our competitors provide us with a major advantage."

In summary, although there are an increasing number of nonclinical roles that physicians play in the health care industry, access to the still limited number of positions is becoming increasingly selective. Despite the many obstacles physicians face in making a transition to the business world, it can be done. Industry insiders give this advice:

▼ Get additional formal training to increase your marketability.

▼ Increase your "industry awareness" (eg, follow the stock market and read major business publications on a regular basis).

▼ If you are interested in R&D, gain a deeper understanding of the Food and Drug Administration's processes.

▼ Convert your curriculum vitae into a resume that translates your work experiences in medicine into language that makes sense to those who hire in the business world.

▼ Be flexible and willing to go back to the bottom of the career ladder as a transitional step. You have to pay your dues all over again.

▼ Be willing to face rejection in your transition, as you surely will encounter a lot of it. (It takes the average industry executive nearly one year to find a new job. It takes the average physician clinician approximately two to three years to cross over to another industry.)

▼ Be humble.

▼ Be tenacious and optimistic. Believe that you can do it. If you hang in there and really go for it, you will eventually succeed.

◢ The Information Technology Market

Of all the new market sectors, perhaps the most interesting one to observe from a development perspective is that of information technology. This sector represents the "Wild, Wild West" in health care.

The IT industry, as a whole, does not have regulatory bodies that function like those in other areas of the health care market (eg, Joint Commission on Accreditation of Healthcare Organizations, National Committee for Quality Assurance, or the Food and Drug Administration). As a result, this business lacks significant standards and regulatory processes at the clinical interface—at least for the moment. The health care IT industry is new enough in its evolution, too, that many hiring authorities admit that physicians represent an especially challenging group of potential employees because it is not clear how to:

▼ take full advantage of their professional expertise,

▼ define optimal selection criteria for hiring them, or

▼ provide the training and support necessary to ensure a successful transition into a nonclinical work setting.

Many of these individuals recall physicians who were hired, only to leave within a year or so because—for one reason or another—"the fit was bad."

From the perspective of physicians as end-users, IT companies are very frustrated that the physician market is so slow to adopt the use of their technology and the Internet. The tendency is to conclude that physicians are simply a change-resistant, technophobic bunch.

The truth is more likely to lie within the less-than-optimal user interfaces and ineffective implementation strategies for IT products and Internet-based tools rather than within the psychodynamics of physician behavior. Major factors slowing down IT adoption by physicians include the complexity of the clinical practice environment and work flow processes, combined with inadequate physician input into product design and implementation strategies.

There is, however, a growing recognition by the IT industry of some of the unique challenges associated with the clinical practice environment. For example, through a special project carried out by anthropologists who spent time observing and "shadowing" physicians in their clinical practices, Intel has gained valuable insights into the complexity of this market.

In fact, as greater insights are gained into the needs of patients and clinicians, the pace of change in health care IT is accelerating rapidly. For example, in mid-1998 Intel coined the term *e-health*. This effectively created the desired "buzz" about the Internet among physicians and patients, and it provides an interesting illustration of the power of a skillful, aggressive public relations campaign in changing attitudes and behaviors across an industry.

MD IntelliNet is being contacted by a rapidly growing number of physicians who have developed their own "homespun" software and Internet-based applications to meet their practice needs. We also strongly encourage many of our physician clients to become more involved in IT-related committees within their hospitals and HMOs as a means of becoming more aware of trends in this market. Indeed, while computers used to be seen as a marginalized area of the medical field, occupied primarily by "nerds," they are now moving into the mainstream culture of the profession. Careers that combine computers and clinical medicine are becoming highly desirable.

Because the need for better collaboration between clinicians and the IT sector is so urgently needed and because the momentum is growing so rapidly, we are likely to see more changes occur in IT than in other health care market sectors. Infusing the clinician perspective more effectively into the IT development and implementation processes will be key to its successful and rapid penetration of the physician market. This has exciting implications for increasing the range and number of career opportunities for physicians interested in this market sector.

◗ Physicians as "Thought Leaders"

It used to be that physicians who performed well during their residency and fellowships made the choice either to remain in academia, where they would generally make less money but stay involved in teaching and research alongside of their clinical activities, or to move into a community-based practice, where they would have less diverse professional activities and experiences but a significantly more lucrative income. Several trends have emerged in the current health care market that relate to this previous career dichotomy. Because of financial pressures on academic institutions today, physicians in teaching hospitals have much less opportunity to teach and do research and are under greater pressures to see more patients. Thus, some now feel they have the *worst* of both worlds—the lack of diversity and intellectual stimulation and the productivity demands typical of private practice, along with the lower compensation of an academic.

In the past, physicians in academia were considered "thought leaders," or "opinion leaders," in the eyes of industry. These were the individuals called upon by companies for expert opinions and to be spokespeople for their products. They were also those targeted by initial marketing campaigns for new products because the so-called influence cascade necessary for a successful product launch began with them. This marketing model is changing in several ways.

In the current marketplace, many companies no longer value the views of academic physicians as much as in the past. They feel these physicians tend to be too narrow and focus too much on the science behind a product. These companies have redefined the concept of thought leader. The new thought leaders may be relegated to providing a perspective where science is balanced by practical business and policy considerations. "The thought leader in today's market has an interest in, and knowledge about, commercial factors. They tend to be more practical and intuitive about medical products. They may, for example, follow the stock market," observes one industry executive.

Physicians in academia tend to be more insulated from business forces within health care, whereas their colleagues in private practice must deal head-on with marketplace realities on a daily basis. Thus, not only do many academicians lack an intuitive and practical sense about health care as business, they also lack a perspective that would be representative of their colleagues in private practice.

For industry, trusting the input of academicians exclusively can be a risky proposition. One investment banking firm I spoke with claimed to have the largest network of physician consultants on contract—to help evaluate potential investment opportunities within the health care industry. "We have a network of 150 physician consultants, and they *all* come from top academic institutions. We believe we are rapidly becoming *the* healthcare investment firm because of this resource pool," they proudly claimed. Yet some in business and medicine alike would question the long-term success of a strategy so exclusively committed to academic medicine.

Physicians in private practice, on the other hand, may well be more able to provide a business-savvy perspective on new products. But they tend not to have the national visibility and name recognition as their academic peers, who publish frequently and speak widely on their research at national conferences.

In addition, the power of the old thought leader has been diluted by the realities of today's health care market. As more and more physicians become integrated into larger organizational entities, their voice in purchasing decisions has become one among many. For example, payers, patients, and employers all have influence on purchasing decisions today. And there is much to suggest that, in the future, the role of consumers in health care financing and decision making will continue to grow, largely due to the success to date of the $3 billion per year spent on direct-to-consumer marketing.[2]

Furthermore, Ed Erickson of the 3M Corporation makes an interesting observation. As the culture of medicine becomes more team oriented and less isolated, he believes that forces of influence upon physicians are being fundamentally altered. "Traditionally, physicians were primarily influenced by where they were trained." He notes that it was quite simple in the past to trace their philosophies, rather like

---

[2] Coddington DC, Moore KD, Fischer EA, Clarke RL. *Beyond Managed Care: The Growing Role of Consumers and Technology.* San Francisco, Calif: Jossey-Bass Publishers. In press.

family lineage, back to their training institutions. He further notes that as the culture evolves, physicians are increasingly being influenced through peer-to-peer collaboration in respected professional circles. Thus their original views learned during training are reshaped over time. This, too, dilutes the power of traditional, academically based "thought leaders."

These changes do not come without significant implications:

▼ Pharmaceutical and medical device companies are rethinking what types of physicians within the clinical services sector can provide the greatest value in obtaining valid market intelligence, influencing their peers, and legitimizing their products to the medical community.

▼ In the IT sector, there is no past generation of physician thought leaders. They are grappling with how to transfer the influence cascade model to new product launches in their sector.

▼ Academic physicians may well be losing market value as it relates to some industry consulting roles previously held by thought leaders.

Although the pendulum is swinging toward increased consumer influence over health care spending, patients still look to their physicians for guidance on most major decisions in their medical care. For this reason, physicians remain an important component of the purchasing engine in the industry.

For physicians interested in transitioning their careers into health care marketing and sales, key trends in the industry to follow include:

▼ the growth of direct-to-consumer marketing,

▼ the emergence of new peer-to-peer marketing models, and

▼ the increasing importance of the Internet as a marketing medium.

▷ Physicians as Entrepreneurs

Most companies involved in new product development for the health care industry receive an overwhelming number of unsolicited ideas from physicians with a product idea. Occasionally these ideas represent viable commercial opportunities, but most of the time they do not.

In addition, most companies spend a substantial amount of time and resources screening these ideas and managing relationships with the physicians who supply them. As industry leaders describe these experiences and individuals, more traits of the cultural impairment syndrome emerge:

▼ Physicians are greedy and have unrealistic expectations about returns on their idea. They think the idea alone entitles them to 99% of any revenues made on eventual product sales.

▼ They have no idea of the complexity of the commercialization process and the resources required.

▼ They have a naive view of industry—huge royalties, brief time to market, pure profit. And they believe no one else has any good ideas.

▼ They are unwilling to share any risk in terms of time, energy, and money.

▼ They want everyone else to do the hard work and want only to reap the rewards.

One executive discussed at length his concern about the increasing number of physician entrepreneurs who "ride the middle." These individuals are trying to supplement their declining incomes from clinical practice by becoming stakeholders in early-stage products being developed for their specialty.

He expressed deep concern about the potential for conflict of interest in these situations, referring to recent experience with a company known as Heartport, Inc. Heartport commercialized a minimally invasive surgical procedure (an alternative to open heart surgery) developed by several physicians at Stanford University. *The Wall Street Journal* reported that the Stanford physicians came under criticism for having a financial interest in the company, even as they were testing its surgical procedure on patients.[3]

One of the executives interviewed clearly has spent a great deal of time thinking about physicians with ideas and how his company should evaluate both the physician and his or her idea. He even has developed a set of "subtypes" applicable to physician entrepreneurs—and designed to help others within his company more easily categorize and triage prospects submitted by physicians. Examples include "The CV Builder," whose primary interest is to add more patents/papers to his list of accomplishments; "The Scientist," whose interest in a product is to satisfy his personal curiosity rather than its successful commercial development; and "The Half & Half," who is half doctor and half entrepreneur. The latter wants to eat his cake (cash in on his idea) and have it too (not assume risk by giving up his practice).

That may seem like unnecessary stereotyping; but certain themes *do* emerge in terms of desirable—and unusual—attributes of physician entrepreneurs, at least as seen through the eyes of potential industry partners/sponsors.

▼ Good ability to communicate

▼ Flexible working and negotiation style

▼ Willingness to roll up their sleeves and actively participate in the development and commercialization process—including giving talks, writing/publishing papers, traveling, and talking with peers about the product

---

[3] King R. Keyhole heart surgery arrived with fanfare, but was it premature? *Wall Street Journal.* May 5, 1999:1, A10.

▼ Clinical credibility

▼ Good understanding of the business context of the product (competitive and marketing issues in particular)

▼ Willingness to share the risk (time, energy, and financial)

In addition, certain types of ideas are more likely than others to generate industry interest. Those where a prototype has been developed or those with a clinical and/or sales history are, of course, the most desirable. In addition, patented ideas, or the work of inventors with visibility and name recognition, also are ideal.

According to research done by Bruce Bornstein, MD, MBA, entrepreneurship among physicians in academic centers could be greatly facilitated by a number of factors that encourage individual initiative.[4]

▼ Increased *availability of mentors and role models* with industry experience.

▼ Establishment of an *academic track for physicians interested in entrepreneurship,* which allows for reduced patient care and general academic responsibilities. These individuals would participate in seminars and other events and would in turn teach the process of commercialization and entrepreneurship to other members of the local academic medical community. One such model exists in the Health Care Entrepreneurship Program at Boston University.

▼ *Efficient technology transfer processes.*

▼ *Clear, unintimidating conflict of interest policies at their institutions of employment.*

▼ Increased *availability of university venture funds* that are separate and remote from mainstream venture capital.

There is no question that physicians in the current market are demonstrating an increased interest in entrepreneurship and are taking more of a leadership role toward that end. One executive commented that, in the past, it was not uncommon to receive calls from academic physicians who were working on a new product idea through their organization's technology transfer office. The callers were interested in finding an industry partner for further R&D and commercialization. Now, however, it is not uncommon for the same type of academic researcher to contact the company about an idea and then call back several weeks later with a new venture already set up to develop and commercialize the product.

---

[4] Bornstein BA. *Commercializing University Biomedical Ideas: Problems and Opportunities* [master's thesis]. Boston, Mass: Massachusetts Institute of Technology; 1999.

◮ Partnerships Across the Great Divide

As traditional funding sources within medicine become more difficult to access, more innovative partnerships are being formed between clinical service organizations and industry (eg, manufacturing firms or investors). Many of these partnerships are still at early stages of development, so it is difficult to assess their long-term success. In addition, many initiatives that have been launched are not highly visible outside their local community, thus making it difficult to identify and learn about them.

This is unfortunate because, as financial pressures throughout the health care industry intensify, it is likely that more and more of these partnerships could prove fruitful for all stakeholders. It also would be an ideal situation if we could collectively leverage past experiences to refine medical/industrial models developed in the future.

Clearly, there are formidable challenges to establishing successful partnerships between clinical service organizations and business entities. One of tremendous concern to many again relates to potential conflicts of interest for physicians who continue to care for patients while having a financial stake in how those patients are managed. A recent article about physicians paid handsomely by pharmaceutical companies to recruit patients into clinical trials illustrates this well.[5] Another article describes a similar potential conflict relating to the referral of cardiac patients to a special cardiac hospital owned by staff physicians.[6]

Another challenge relates to negative or narrow attitudes that one camp holds about the other. One industry-based physician described the discussions that took place about a potential new clinical research partnership between a network of hospitals and a major pharmaceutical company. "As we tried to set the program up it became clear that the academic department chiefs held some very arrogant attitudes about what pharmaceutical companies had to offer them," he recounts. The academics believed they had cornered the market on intellectual capital and research methodology. Industry, they believed, had little more to offer the initiative than money. There was no consideration of intellectual partnership and no consideration that the company's research might be at least as good as that done within academia. Their ideas were so firmly fixed, and there was so much resistance to any productive dialogue, that further discussion about the potential partnership ceased.

Although there are a number of potential barriers to forming such partnerships, some initiatives have worked through the challenging initial discussion stage to a successful launch. Here are five notable examples:

---

[5] Eichenwald E, Kolata G. Drug trials hide conflicts for doctors. *New York Times.* May 16, 1999:1, 28-29.

[6] Winslow R. Fed-up cardiologists invest in own hospital just for heart disease. *Wall Street Journal.* June 22, 1999:1, A12.

▼ 3M Corporation and the Mayo Clinic have recently formed an alliance in which a 3M fund provides grants for programs proposed by co-investigators from each institution. The proposals target defined therapeutic areas and are reviewed by a peer review committee composed of individuals from each institution.

▼ The Clinical Research Institute (CRI) is a community-based, university-affiliated program that conducts clinical research for the pharmaceutical industry. The program was established by a physician (Ronald E. Keeney, MD) with 22 years of experience in that industry. During this time, he was frequently disappointed in the quality of study sites and the lack of understanding of what constitutes a good clinical practice research model.

CRI was set up at WakeMed, a community-based hospital affiliated with the University of North Carolina at Chapel Hill and located near Research Triangle Park. CRI strategically capitalizes on the high-quality resources of the academic center, the primary care patient base of the community hospital and its referral network, and Dr Keeney's extensive industry experience. In addition, CRI provides interested medical students and residents with a rich training opportunity in clinical research.

▼ In 1997 Genzyme Corporation and Partners HealthCare System, Inc, Boston's largest medical care organization, formed an alliance to collaborate on a broad range of scientific research and clinical trials. Although it is not uncommon for hospitals and drug companies to form partnerships, they usually focus on specific diseases and therapies. This one, which crosses over 10 specialty areas, is unusual for its breadth.

▼ The Massachusetts General Hospital (MGH)/Harvard Cutaneous Biology Research Center (CBRC) was established in 1989 by a multiyear contract between MGH and Shiseido Co (a Tokyo-based cosmetics company) to conduct dermatological research in molecular and cellular biology. To date, the company has provided $180 million of research support and has maintained its commitment to uphold the academic freedom of the 12 principal investigators and 50 research fellows to pursue research topics of their choice within dermatology.

▼ The University of Texas Medical Branch at Galveston teamed with the Teletraining Institute in Stillwater, Oklahoma, to create the Open Gates Teletraining Institute in 1997. This venture positions itself as a leader in education on the "distance-bridging" technology in health care.

All of the above represent examples of partnerships that provide academically based or affiliated physicians with a broader range of career opportunities. However, physicians based in nonacademic clinical settings are beginning to see expanded career opportunities as well. For example, physicians in practices associated with PhyMatrix Corporation and Universal Health Services, Inc, now have greater access to clinical research participation through their partnership with Clinical Studies, Ltd, a site management organization (SMO).

It is likely that more partnerships will form between the clinical and business sides of the health care industry in coming years. Given that the goal of industry in most of these partnerships is access to a large number of physicians and patients, physicians affiliated with large entities are likely to be at an advantage. That's one potential consolation for those grieving the loss of their small, independent practice.

◣ Concluding Thoughts

The rapid pace of change and complex challenges presented by the current health care marketplace also create unprecedented opportunities for collaboration between industry and the medical profession. Such collaborations have never been easy to structure or manage. Success requires creating workable, productive interactions between two very different cultures. In addition, there must be constant vigilance against potential conflicts of interest and maintenance of impeccable ethical standards.

That said, there are vast and exciting possibilities for creative and valuable collaboration between the worlds of clinical medicine and business. These are limited only by an unwillingness to reconsider long-held negative assumptions and biases each group holds toward the other. In the current context of change, those who choose not to step back and reflect on their own constraining beliefs will be at an increasing disadvantage.

References

Blumenthal D. Ethics issues in academic-industry relationships in the life sciences: the continuing debate. *Acad Med.* 1996;71:1291-1296.

Blumenthal D. Growing pains for new academic/industry relationships. *Health Aff 13.* 1994;No. 3:176-193.

Brett AM, Bibson DV, Smilor RW, eds. *University Spin-Off Companies: Economic Development, Faculty Entrepreneurs and Technology Transfer.* Savage, Md: Rowman & Littlefield; 1991.

Dorf RC, Worthington KKF. Technology transfer: research to commercial product. *Eng Manage Int.* 1989;5:185-191.

Nelson L. Essays on science and society: the rise of intellectual property protection in the American university. *Sci Magazine.* 1998;279:1460-1461.

Ono RD, ed. *The Business of Biotechnology: From the Bench to the Street.* Stoneham, Mass: Butterworth-Heineman; 1991.

Roberts EB. *Entrepreneurship in High Technology: Lessons from MIT and Beyond.* New York, NY: Oxford University Press; 1991.

Roberts EB, Malone DE. Policies and structures for spinning off new companies from research and development organizations. *R&D Manage 26.* 1996;No. 1:17-48.

Salemi T. Medical schools forming funds to plug seed gap. *Venture Capital and Health Care 3.* Wellesley, Mass: Asset Alternatives; 1999;No. 3:1, 25, 26.

Chapter 9

Envisioning Your Future

Given all the time, energy, and money invested in your education, it's a downright travesty there is no good career guidance model for those who want to pursue medicine. Misguided decisions could be minimized through a better system of career guidance *throughout* one's training. Indeed, it is becoming clear that the lack of early and ongoing career counseling represents a fundamental flaw in medical education as it currently exists.

Higher education, especially in medicine, understandably encourages students to focus their interests and learning. This results in more expertise, which for the most part serves medicine well. It does come at a cost, though—a cost that is taking a substantial toll on individual physicians *and* the profession as a whole.

The insular nature of physicians' training limits their awareness of career diversification and growth opportunities. It also limits their access to those outside of medicine—and their ability to effectively communicate, collaborate, and negotiate with them.

◢ Envisioning Your *Individual* Future

Your medical career needs to be *actively* managed. You must maintain awareness of the world around clinical medicine, which influences and shapes it each day.

Start by reading nonprofessional daily and monthly publications. This can be challenging, given the information needed just to stay on top of your specialty. It's easier if you subscribe to those publications that screen a range of sources to deliver only what's of special interest to you.

Again, the Internet can play a vital role because of its ability to filter even the most arcane subject matter for a daily dose of news, such as three-dimensional computer software that may apply to your avocation as a programmer as well as to your neurology specialty.

Keep up with your colleagues—nonphysicians as well as physicians. An active network allows you to build the bridge for your next career stage, even if it's far into the future. Remain aware of how we physicians are perceived by our colleagues in the business world. Make an effort to modify those behaviors that, however appropriate within a clinical medicine setting, are clearly counterproductive to your career diversification goals.

◆ Envisioning Our *Collective* Future

We have a collective responsibility as physicians to help those who follow us avoid all the trials and tribulations that have plagued medicine toward the end of the 20th century. There are a number of things we can do—as members of medical societies, hospital medical staffs, HMO panels, etc.

Ensure that good career guidance exists at all stages of medical education. We should not leave such counseling to the province of medical faculty because they are biased toward academia and have little or no knowledge of professional life outside the Ivory Tower.

We need to help young people make their medical career decisions for the *right* reasons. Too many physicians are misguided in their choice of medicine. They may have misconceptions about the profession. They may enter the field because it was "expected" of them or because they're "good in science."

In these cases, it would take very little in the way of objective evaluation or discussion to help an undergraduate, medical student, or resident see that medicine (or a specific subset, say clinical vs research, or pediatrics vs pathology) may *not* be the best path for them. On the other hand, this early intervention in the selection process could reinforce that the student's decision is right. This in itself can be extremely valuable. This service should be provided for *all* trainees—a requisite included in the cost of tuition.

There needs to be acceptance and support of more flexible work models within clinical medicine. It is important that physicians have the option to work full- or part-time, whether it be to enhance work-life balance or to pursue diversification activities. At present, this option is limited for a number of reasons (eg, credentialing policies, attitudes within the profession, lack of practical models). We need to do all we can to facilitate and legitimize part-time clinical work as an option for *all* physicians.

We must become activists and role models if we are to expand the presence of physicians in business. If physicians effectively play a broader range of roles throughout health care, it stands to benefit the entire industry.

Physicians who combine their MD degree with equivalent business skills can provide a voice too often missing in the ongoing power struggle. This is an issue of diversity—physicians are still a minority in industry. As we have more and more contact and successful relationships with that culture, we can break down the barriers that divide us.

It is hard for physicians interested in career diversification or transition to find a mentor—even for one-time advice. Recognizing this, MD IntelliNet's Web site (www.mdintellinet.com) includes (with permission) case studies and e-mail addresses of physician clients who have made such transitions. Web site visitors report these vignettes to be among its most valuable features, primarily because they've never before known actual examples of physician transitions to industry.

We need to make more visible the exciting and successful partnerships between industry and provider organizations—both within and outside of academia. We need to build on these models and leverage what we learn from each.

The profession needs to launch an aggressive public relations campaign to improve the image of physicians in the eyes of industry. Many physicians make very successful transitions. These stories need more play in the media.

We need more cross-disciplinary training and diverse hands-on experiences for medical students, residents, and mid-career clinicians. Making these opportunities part of their ongoing education legitimizes a broader range of career options.

Managed care has created exquisite pain and uncertainty within the medical profession. We have been forced to reflect upon our roles, relationships, and identity within the health care industry. Unquestionably, some of these reflections are associated with a great sense of angst, sadness, and anger about what American medicine has lost in all the turmoil. Managed care did indeed mark the end of an era for the medical profession.

On further reflection, however, it also becomes possible to see the potential for *growth*—on both the individual and collective level. As our *professional* development becomes integrated with *career* development, many possibilities emerge.

Strategic career management for the 21st century physician opens up the prospect of:

▼ creating healthy, balanced lives for physicians within our personal, professional, and organizational spheres;

▼ ongoing growth and development *throughout* our careers;

▼ improving the quality of care for our patients;

▼ expanding our sphere of influence beyond the bedside within the health care industry;

▼ greater opportunities for physician participation in innovation; and

▼ realizing our full potential to contribute at each stage of our careers.

> *What we call the beginning is often the end*
> *And to make an end is to make a beginning.*
> *The end is where we start from.*[1]

---

[1] Eliot TS. *Little Gidding.* New York, NY: Harcourt, Brace; 1943:38.

Index